The GREATTASTIC ADVENTURES: Miracle Child

J. Mitchell Ulibarri

"Do I not destroy my enemies when I make them my friends?"

-Abraham Lincoln

I have changed some names, locations, and details to protect individuals' privacy. These are my memories from my perspective, or in some cases information I received in doing research for this book. I have tried to represent events as accurately as possible.

To request permissions, contact the publisher at rules4agreattasticlife@gmailcom

ISBN: 9781637951552

Ebook ISBN: 9781637951569

ICCN:2021902305

First paperback edition April 2021

Edited by Luke Ulibarri, Joshua Ulibarri, Sandra Ulibarri, Leela Ramey, Ryan Ulibarri, and Amy Carney
Cover art by: Hope Hinger and Kobolt Design Studios Inc.
Layout by: Kindle Direct Publishing

Printed by Kindle Direct Publishing in the USA.

John Mitchell Ulibarri
P.O. Box 14443 Columbus, OH 43214

TABLE OF CONTENTS

ACKNOWLEDGEMENTS

Many thanks to Luke, Josh, Mom, Dad, Leela, Ryan, and Mrs. Carney for helping me edit this book, and thank you Hope and Kobolt Design Studios, Inc. for the cover art.

SEASON 1: A FRIENDSHIP GONE BAD

AUTHOR'S NOTE

Autism is a learning disability found in people all over the world. As you may know from my blog and podcast, I have autism. Because of autism, I have always had trouble making friends. It's not that I didn't understand all the social cues, though that was part of the problem. The main issue was that in school, I was bullied a lot. As a result, if anyone did anything that hurt me, I immediately assumed they were just as bad. This assumption caused the problem I ran into with the girls. While they are my "sisters" now, it took years to get to this point. The Anderson girls have been there for me since this book's events had first begun, and I love each of them dearly.

When I first started my blog, I wrote an article called "Not Just Black And White." It was about the fight that began the mutual contempt between the girls and me. Because I was planning on writing this book, I had to leave out some details. The girls thought that they came out looking bad. I honestly don't think they did, but to each his own. The big reason I didn't believe it was too big of a deal at the time was because of this book. This book explains how We became friends and why it was so hard for us to get to that point. August, Arden, Aspen, and Arlo - this is for you.

Hope you enjoy and Have a Greattastic Day,
J. Mitchell Ulibarri

Disclaimer: Some names and places have been changed for the privacy of the characters.

Dedication

I am writing this book for my Nimba, my parents, and my brothers Ryan, Luke, and Josh for supporting me no matter what, for Samantha McCarthy (my best friend), for the rest of my family, and of course (as already mentioned) for the Anderson girls.

PROLOGUE: THE PROJECT
01/05/2011

I looked out the window and froze. August and Arden were walking around "the circle." I knew what I had to do. I had been planning it all day, but August would make things difficult. I ran to the front door and onto my porch as fast as I could. The cold wind took my breath away. As I was composing myself, the door slammed behind me, and the girls looked up.

"Hey, guys!" I said, but they did not respond. I walked down the stairs, through the frost-covered grass onto the street, and started walking next to them. "How are you?" I asked, still with no reply. I stood in front of them and took a deep breath, "Okay. I know we don't get along anymore, but I need your help."

"What?" they both asked in utter confusion.

I proposed my idea: "I have this school project."

"What is it?" Arden asked hesitantly.

"I have to make a movie."

"No! Absolutely not!" August responded immediately, making it seem as if her life depended on it.

"Come on!" I pleaded. "I know you have made videos with Shelby."

"Well," Arden said, "she has never attacked us. We can't trust you."

"I can earn your trust."

"Really?" the girls asked together.

"Yes," I replied with confidence.

"We have to talk to the girls," August said,

3

referring to her other sisters as she turned into their driveway.

"Come with us," Arden said, walking towards the house.

"You're on thin ice, Mr.!" August said as we walked to their side door. My hands were shaking, and I couldn't believe that this plan had a slight chance of working.

But this is not the beginning of my life with the girls. I wish it were, it would have made things much less stressful. I guess it's a good thing, however, because otherwise, our friendship would not be as strong as it is today. As everyone's stories do, mine begins with my parents meeting.

CHAPTER 1: THE BEST OF FRIENDS
04/19/1915-04/04/1988

Milton Opper was born on April 19th, 1915, in Sandusky, Ohio. He grew up on his family's farm as a member of the Methodist Church. When he was in his twenties, he went out to a party with a friend of his. While they were at this party, they saw two beautiful women. Milt and his friend approached the two women. Milt tapped the one on the left's shoulder; however, the woman on the right thought Milt had touched her.

The woman on the right was a Catholic girl named Laurene Kessler. She would be responsible for Milt's conversion to Catholicism. Milt became a deacon in the church and was active from the age of 58 until he was 101. Laurene and Milt were married and had two kids: Charles and Bev. The kids had a fantastic childhood, and they both made wonderful friends.

When Bev was in high school, she met a man named John Biehl. The summer following their graduation, John and Bev got married. Soon after that, they had three children together: Bob, Sandra, and Melissa.

However, John and Bev had bigger plans for their family. Rather than living in the small town of Sandusky, they moved two hours away to the Columbus area. Bev got a job as an administrative assistant, and John started working his way through law school.

The marriage was not meant to last and ended in divorce. John moved to New York to pursue a job opportunity while Bev and the children stayed in Columbus. A few years after the divorce, Bev met Jack Savage. Bev and Jack got married and had two daughters: Shana and Cyndi. That is how the Biehl/Savage family came to be. Sandra grew up and went to school at The Ohio State University for interior design. Little did she know that her life was about to change forever:

"Mom, I got the job!" Sandra said to her mom over the phone.

"That's great, honey! When do you start?"

"Next week!"

"Have you told Tom?"

"Well--" Sandra started, just as her roommate ran into the dorm.

"San!" her roommate exclaimed, "You have to come outside! I met this cool guy. You have to meet him!"

"Hey Mom, Shannon wants me to meet someone. I'll call you back!"

"Okay, love you!"

"Love you too!"

Sandra and Shannon went outside. Sandra started asking about the guy. He was a student from the Columbus College of Art and Design, and his name was Jerry. Jerry was about average height with dark brown curly hair and stubble all over his face. He also drove a captivating green MGB.

Sandra and Jerry hit it off right away. There were no awkward pauses. They made each other laugh, they

6

were both Catholic, and they had similar views about the negative effects of divorce, as Jerry came from a similar situation to Sandra.

"San," Shannon said when Jerry had left. "What about Tom?"

"About that," Sandra said, "I broke up with him last night--"

Shannon cheered because she knew Sandra was way too good for Tom. Sandra and Jerry hung out a lot that week, and by the end of it, they were a couple.

The job Sandra got was at a daycare center. On her first day, she walked into the classroom, not knowing what to expect. It was a room full of kids and only one adult supervisor. Sandra introduced herself to the supervisor just as another woman walked into the room.

"Sandra," the supervisor said, "this is Anita, my other assistant!"

As the day went on, Sandra and Anita started to get to know each other. At one point or another, Sandra told Anita about how she had just started dating Jerry. They discovered that Anita's long-time boyfriend, Ron, was also going to school at the Columbus College of Art and Design.

And with that, a new age began. Sandra, Jerry, Anita, and Ron became best friends and remain that way to this day. Both couples ended up getting married, bought their first homes and within a few years, they all had kids.

CHAPTER 2: THE BIRTH OF RYAN
02/05/1995-01/14/2000

The parking lot outside of the art firm in Columbus was covered in a blanket of snow. Jerry opened the door, and a cold wind rushed in. He started his long trudge to his car as snow filled his shoes. After what felt like years, Jerry jumped in his car and hit the road. He got stuck in rush hour traffic, so it took him about an hour to get home to Clintonville.

"Finally!" he said, turning off the car when he got home. "Now," he said to himself as he walked to the door, "I have to tell San." As if on cue, the back door opened, and Sandra stood in the doorway.

"Hi," she said when he came in. "How was your day… what's wrong?"

"I think I have to quit my job," he replied as he walked into the kitchen.

"What!"

"The company is moving to New York. We can move and start over in a new place, or we can stay here and keep building our lives. We already have a start here. Your family is here, and all our friends are here. We need to stay here!"

Neither Sandra nor Jerry wanted to move to New York. They felt Jerry had a lot of good connections in the industry in Columbus, so this would be a good opportunity to start a business of their own.

"Starting a new business, it is a big risk. So many things could go wrong. What if you try and it doesn't work?" All the typical questions swirled around in their minds.

"It will work. We will make it work!" Jerry said. She trusted him and his ability to run a business.

They were right in doing so. Almost immediately, "Kobolt Design Studios" was a steady income source for Sandra and Jerry. They were enjoying their lives and did some traveling with Anita and Ron.

They were pleasantly surprised when they found out they were pregnant with me: John Mitchell Ulibarri. I was born on August 19, 1997. Soon after I was brought home from the hospital, Becca, the little girl who lived next door, started spending a lot of time with me. She was an only child, and it was convenient because we could play in our backyard and we got along really well.

I had this little green turtle sandbox, where Becca and I spent all our time. Whenever I would see her, I would start flapping my hands and squealing because I was excited. I would often make up stories with her using the sand in the sandbox.

When I was around three years old, I was obsessed with the Nickelodeon show, *Blue's Clues*. I had all of Steve's shirts, a Handy Dandy Notebook, and even my own Thinking Chair! When Becca and I weren't outside in the sandbox, we were inside my house watching Blue's Clues, or playing a game that we called "chase," which was basically tag. That was what my life was like for the first few years, but everything changed when Mom and Dad were expecting my little brother. From the start, they

9

knew we would eventually have to move off of the busy street we lived on and into a bigger house.

When I was little, I couldn't say grandma, so I called Bev "Nimba," and the name stuck. I remember Nimba taking me to the hospital one cold January day, and from that point forward, my life was changed forever.

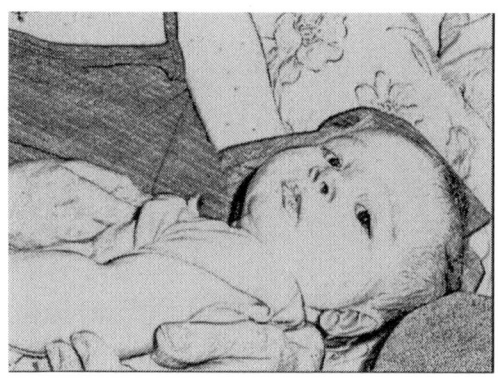

"Mitchell," Mom said from the hospital bed, "this is your brother Ryan." I climbed up on the hospital bed and sat next to Mom, so I could see. In her arms was a small baby with a tuft of brown hair, and a small vein on his forehead. I reached out to touch him.

"Be careful, Mitchell!" Dad warned. I took my finger and touched Ryan inquisitively. Immediately, he opened his brown eyes.

"Look," Mom said, "He likes you," and with that, I was in love. After about 10-15 minutes, a nurse came into the room and took Ryan.

"NO!" I yelled at the nurse when she started to walk away.

"What's wrong?" Mom asked, taken aback.

"SHE'S TAKING HIM AWAY!" I exclaimed as tears ran down my cheeks. My parents looked at each other, awed by my confusion and my immediate connection to Ryan.

"I'll bring him right back," the nurse said with a smile.

"You promise?"

"Yes, I promise," she assured me. "You're going to be a great big brother!"

For the next few months, Becca and I would play with Ryan. Well, I say "play with"; mostly, we would play *next* to him. That was my life until we moved when I was almost four years old.

CHAPTER 3: THE FAIRYTALE
06/01/2001

We moved onto a street called Meadow Park Drive. Meadow Park was a hill with "The Circle" at the bottom. To the right of "The Circle" was a small street leading back out to the main road called Meadow Park Place. Behind "The Circle" were three houses. On the right was a white house that belonged to a newlywed couple. On the left was a yellow house behind an enormous pine tree belonging to Rich and Barbara Anderson, who had three girls. In between those houses was a brick house now owned by my family.

My house had five rooms on the main floor: kitchen, living room, TV room, and two dining rooms. The kitchen had a white tile floor, chrome appliances, and some shelves which were being built by Dad. The living room had a massive mantle with a muppet-like creature engraved into the wood right above the fireplace. To the left of the mantle was a space that someday would hold a baby grand piano. All of the rooms were completely furnished.

I remember being upset the day we moved because I missed Becca; however, I would soon forget my problems. Mom went outside later that day with Ryan. Not wanting to be alone in the house, I followed. She walked to the circle. "The Circle" is an island in the middle of the street named after its shape. The outer circle is filled with grass, eight trees, and other plant life. The inner circle, however, has three wooden benches on a paver covered ground. The trees block the sun making a peaceful spot for people to relax.

Mom sat on one of the benches, and I ran as fast as I could to get to her. Before I even had made it out of my driveway Barbara walked out of hers.

"Hi, Barbara," Mom called.

"Hello, Sandra," Barbara replied, "All moved in?"

"As much as we'll ever be."

"And who is this?" she asked, pointing to Ryan.

"This is Ryan, and that's Mitchell." Mom said pointing to me as I walked up behind Barbara.

"Oh!" said Barbara, turning on her heel. "Hi Mitchell. I'm Barbara. How old are you?"

"Three!" I said proudly.

"I have a couple of daughters who are around your age!"

"Really?" I asked.

"Yep. One is four, and the other is three. Both are inside, do you want to go meet them?"

"Okay!" I said, excited to meet more new people.

We walked through the front door into the house and into the living room. It had a long couch and a chair facing a fireplace. I walked around the house finding the kitchen/dining room, sunroom, and the "guest" dining room looping back to the living room. As I walked, I noticed many pictures of Jesus, Mary, and other religious figures hanging on the walls. I also noticed small angel statues had been placed all over. When I entered the living room for the second time, I realized a little piano was pushed up against the wall.

Now, Nimba happened to have a piano. Whenever we would go to her house for a family gathering, I would have a concert. I didn't know how to play it, of course. I would just very aggressively pound on the keys. So, when I saw the piano that day, my first instinct was to "play."

As I got up on the piano bench a girl with long brown hair, blue eyes, and freckles walked out from an opening in the wall that I hadn't noticed.

"Mommy?" she called as I brought my fists down on the piano. She jumped and froze when she saw me.

"Hi!" I said. "I'm Mitchell."

"I'm Arden. My sister is in the other room," she said, walking back into the room she had come from. I followed her and saw another girl with similar characteristics, sitting on a brown couch in front of a TV. A look of shock descended upon her face when I walked into the room because of my sudden arrival.

"Mitchell," Arden said, "this is August, my big sister."

"Hi," she said hesitantly.

"Hello!" I replied. A silence that would never be heard in that house again fell, and I took my chance. "You want to play a game?" I asked.

"What game?" asked Arden.

"Chase!"

"What's that?" August asked.

"It's a game my friend Becca and I play."

"How does it--" but before August could finish her sentence, I jumped on the couch. August jumped off the couch, and she and Arden ran out of the room. We ran and giggled around the house without a care in the world. We reached the sunroom, and I happened to look out of the sliding glass door at the back of the house and Mom and Barbara were now in the backyard. The sight before me was astonishing. The Andersons' backyard was an endless, magical forest. The trees stood hundreds of feet high in the air, and there was a playset in a "meadow." A log cabin that I thought belonged to elves stood in the middle of the meadow. To the right side was a giant trampoline. I stood in awe for a few moments until finally I decided to open my mouth to tell the girls how awesome it was. I was about to speak when Arden put her finger over her mouth.

"What?" I asked.

"Uh-oh," August said after hearing *it*.

"We should get Mommy," said Arden. Still confused, I listened until I heard crying. We ran outside and told our moms what had happened. When she heard, Barbara ran inside, followed by me, the girls, and Mom. After a few minutes, she came down holding a baby.

"Who is this?" Mom asked.

"This is Aspen," Barbara replied.

We got a white blanket out and placed both Ryan and Aspen on it. For the next hour, the girls and I played with the babies while both of our moms talked. That was the beginning of our Fairytale Childhood. We spent all of our time together and had many adventures, including:

- Going on trips together
- Going to Mass together
- Switching off who would take the kids every Thursday so that the other couple could have a date night
- Celebrating birthdays
- Having sleepovers
- Learning to play the piano together

15

But as you probably know, even fairytales have problems that the characters need to overcome. A villain who tries to destroy everything that the hero holds dear. Unfortunately, that villain was me, and this fairytale did not end in a "Happily Ever After."

CHAPTER 4: "THE TORTOISE AND THE HARE"

06/24/2005

We had many more adventures during our fairytale childhood. My parents had two more children, Luke and Josh. Barbara and Richard also had one more child, Arlo who was nicknamed Lo-lo, and we all continued to play together. During this time, August and I got "married." All our stuffed animals and imaginary friends showed up; it was a beautiful ceremony.

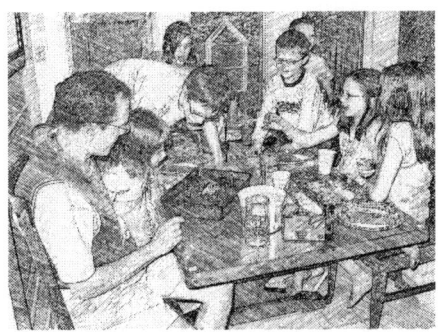

But one of the biggest things we all did together was date night. Barbara and Rich would take care of all eight kids one Thursday so my parents could go on a date. The next Thursday, Mom and Dad took care of the kids.

Every date night we had at the Andersons' house we had pizza. A big reason we had pizza was that I have an aversion to the texture of meat, so pizza makes dinner really easy. After pizza, in an attempt to stop complete insanity from breaking out, Barbara would get out this little wooden train station set for everyone to play with. To be fair, insanity still ensued, but at least she tried.

One time I was late for a date night at the Andersons' house. Everyone else got really excited about playing with the trains. They all shoveled pizza into their mouths and were pretty much done eating by the time I got there. I sat with them for about five minutes before they left.

There I was trying to eat my dinner while my friends and brothers were in the other room having a ton of fun. I started to feel lonely and left out. Eventually, Rich walked into the kitchen. He was a well-dressed man in his mid-40s.

"What's wrong?" he asked when he saw me.

"Nothing."

"Mitchell," he said, sitting down next to me, "are you sure?" I explained the situation and how I was feeling. Without a second of hesitation, he told me the story of "The Tortoise and the Hare." The moral of the story, of course, is "slow and steady wins the race." When the story was finished, I felt a lot better about the situation. My confidence was restored, and I went on with my night. What I didn't realize then was what the friendship Rich and I had started would inevitably become—a mentorship.

CHAPTER 5: THE WORLD ENDS

03/15/2005-07/07/2009

Our fairytale childhood continued without any problems until I was in first grade. You see, the newlywed couple in the white house next to us were expecting a baby. They didn't think the school district was the best, so they put the house up for sale. It was eventually sold to Nate and Liz Parker, who had two kids.

Gregory, their son, was my age, so he befriended me; his sister, Melody, was Aspen's age and became her friend. Greg was small with short brown hair and blue eyes. In all honesty, initially, I didn't get along with Greg. I thought he was a little overbearing, and he thought that the girls were weird, so he would talk trash about them. I was his friend pre-middle school, for three reasons:

1. At this point, I only had six close friends: the Andersons and two girls from school. In other words, Greg was my only friend who was a boy.
2. He introduced me to Star Wars, and we bonded over that.
3. My parents, mostly Mom, encouraged me to be friends with him. "Mitchell," she would say, "he just moved in. He doesn't have any friends around. Just try to be his friend." So, I pursued the friendship.

Mrs. Parker and Dad didn't really get along. Now because of their disagreements, Melody started to dislike Dad, and she would talk to the girls about it.

Around the same time, another family moved in right behind my family. Stephen Crawford was a former soldier in the military and worked for the government. Stephen's wife, Robin, was a nurse. The couple had adopted two girls from China named Megan and Rachel. Our families started hanging out regularly. One day, Stephen was working from home when he heard a shuffling noise coming from the other room. Since his kids were out with Robin, he figured it was a robber. He followed the sound ready to fight an intruder, only to find a four-year-old Aspen sitting on the floor playing with Megan's Barbies.

"You have good toys!" the little girl exclaimed.

"Gahh!" Stephen yelled as he ushered her out of the house.

"Oh, there you are!" said August when Stephen and Aspen exited the house.

"Thank you!" said Arden to Stephen, and the three girls walked off, giggling the whole time. Stephen felt uncomfortable with the situation since he was home alone. Despite the circumstances, the fairytale continued. We still had date night, we played together, and we still had fun doing it.

When I was in second grade, the end finally started. Ryan started kindergarten that year, and on his first day, he met a kid named Brett Lantz. Both Brett and Ryan were shy little kids, so they became best friends within a week. By the end of that year, they had made a few more friends, Mickey Roberts and a pair of twins,

Ross and Mike Young. But when Ryan was in first grade everything changed. That was the year that Will Hoag and Ryan became friends.

Will was just as small as everyone else in Ryan's group. Despite his size, however, Will is the most confident and outgoing person I have ever met. Because of his personality, he has an effect on people. People tend to follow him, and when they are around him, they tend to be excited, energized, or happy in general. Will chose to join Ryan's friend group, became its leader, and named it "The Duck Clan."

Whenever The Duck Clan would hang out, Helen Hoag, Nick Lantz, Luke, Josh, and I would tag along. I started to consider them my school friends because when I was in fourth grade, the amount of bullying I had to endure picked up.

Almost every week in the summer, from when I was in second through fifth grade, my brothers, the girls, and I would have water gun fights. The one constant in these fights was that the girls always won. At first, they won because of strategy, but after a while they got bored. The girls started to, for lack of a better word, cheat. For example, they would bring buckets of water, fill their guns with ice water, steal our weapons, etc. We didn't care about it, though; it was all in good fun.

One day in the summer, between my fifth and sixth grade, Will came over.

"Ryan," Will said when he came in the door, "the neighbor girls are outside, and they want everyone to come out." So, Ryan, Luke, Josh, and Will walked outside. August, Arden, and Aspen were waiting for the boys in the circle.

"Where's Mitchell?" Arden asked when she saw Ryan.

"He's with Greg, playing Mario."

"Typical," said August. "Well, we're hot; let's have a water gun fight." The boys agreed, and it started. At first, everything went as usual. The girls drenched the boys, the boys retreated, and the girls got bored. One of the girls decided it would be fun to add liquid soap to the water. After telling the other girls about the plan, they ran back to their house.

"What's going on?" Luke asked after about a minute.

"I don't know," replied Ryan. "They wouldn't run."

"Come on," Will said, "let's see what they're doing!" As Will led the boys slowly to the front of the house, the girls stalked their prey.

"NOW!" August yelled when the boys were in range. Since Luke and Josh were in the back of the group, they got away swiftly. However, the stream of soapy water hit Will and Ryan. Ryan got some in his mouth and spat it out. Will got shot in the eye and started complaining.

Ryan helped Will into our house and got Mom. She helped clean out Will's bloodshot eye and helped him calm down. When he felt better, Will went to the window. The girls were talking to each other under the pine tree.

"Those girls," Will said, "we need to get back at them!"

"What should we do?" Ryan asked.

"Well, they used soap, so what if we use mud?" The boys really liked the idea, so they walked out to the

22

back and filled their guns with dirt and water. What happened next is unclear. The boys say that they just used the weapons, while the girls claim they threw sticks. Either way, things just went downhill from there.

I walked into my house about an hour after the game had ended. I could hear Dad saying something in a scolding voice. When I asked Mom, she said that Rich had told Dad that Will, Ryan, Luke, and Josh had hurt the girls. After a while, Dad left and started talking to Mom. I slipped away to investigate. I saw Ryan was upset, but he wouldn't tell me what had happened. I looked at Will, and he explained everything. By the time he was finished talking, I was so angry I thought I was going to explode. How could the girls hurt Will and expect him not to retaliate? Why was Dad not feeling the same way I was? Why did the girls want to get my brothers in trouble for something that was their own fault? Why would they want to make Ryan upset? I felt very protective of Ryan and the others and knew that the girls couldn't get away with this!

I stormed outside, looked around, and then I spotted them. August and Arden were talking to each other in front of their house. They were still covered in mud, but they didn't seem to notice me. I ran as fast as I could across the yard, so they didn't see me until I was right on top of them. Arden turned to look at me, confused. I grabbed her and dug my fingernails into her shoulders. Her ice-blue eyes closed, she let out a scream and tears streamed down her cheeks.

Without warning, I was knocked on the ground. I looked up only to see August looking down at me. Her eyes were narrowed, and her face was twisted in anger. I kicked her in the shin and tried to escape. She was faster than me, so I didn't get far. She punched and kicked me until I was on the ground.

"Hey!" Dad yelled, running out the door. "What are you doing!"

"I... I…" August said, caught off guard, "I was defending Arden." I got to my knees and reached for my glasses, which had fallen off my face.

"No, you weren't," I said. "I came outside, and you just started hitting me!"

"No, I didn't! You attacked Arden! You liar!"

"August!" Dad exclaimed. "Mitchell said you just started hitting him and I saw the same thing! I'm going to have to tell your dad!" August glared at me, and I smiled back.

Dad told Rich what had "happened." The girls tried to defend themselves but nothing they said changed Dad's perception. With that, our friendship with the Andersons and the fairytale, our whole world, ended.

My relationship with Greg flourished, as did my family's with Stephen and Robin. Greg and I would do whatever it took to get the girls and Melody in trouble. It was always the same story. We would do something, the girls would retaliate, and I would tell Dad that they were the bad guys. The girls grew to hate my family and me, and this went on and on. Fortunately, there was one last hope that we had. One person who could potentially get us out of this: Arden.

CHAPTER 6: THE PLAN
10/09/2009

I went to a small Catholic grade school attached to my church, Our Lady of Peace (OLP). My kindergarten teacher, Mrs. Smith, left the school when I was in first grade. Because Mrs. Smith left, the half-day Kindergarten teacher took her job. This left the half-day kindergarten without a teacher. The principal, Mrs. Fields hired a woman by the name of Martha Green to run the half-day kindergarten.

I had been bullied throughout the first half of my first-grade year because I was different. After Christmas that year, I befriended a girl named Sam, and she became my best friend. As a result of our friendship, I didn't notice the bullying as much after that. At the end of third grade, unfortunately, her family moved away.

Luckily for me, I did happen to have a couple people to hang out with. One of them was named Alice, and the other was a guy named Pete. Pete was socially awkward, and Alice was a little bigger than the other girls in our class. We bonded because we were the outcasts of our class. There were a few people who hung out with us from time to time. One of Alice's best friends was with us a lot, and there was another boy named Alex, but for the most part, it was just Alice, Pete, and I. Even though I had this friend group, I wasn't able to ignore the bullying. By the time I got to 6th grade the bullying got so bad I would hide in the bathroom to avoid being around the bullies. Eventually of course, this habit caught up with me.

The bell rang at 2:35 PM as it always did, but today was different. It was the last day of the first quarter, and I had just gotten my report card. I could feel my heart frantically jumping around my chest. Ms. Hickman, my sixth-grade teacher, walked out of the classroom with her students closely behind, but I stayed at my desk.

"Cs and Ds," I said to myself. "What am I going to do?" I put my head down and closed my eyes.

"Mitchell Ulibarri," Mrs. Fields called over the loudspeaker, "if you are still in the building, please come to my office." I looked up at the clock. It was 3:10. I stood up, took a deep breath, and started to walk down to the office. Right outside of the office stood Mom, Mrs. Fields, Mrs. Green, Ryan, Luke, and Josh. Mom's arms were crossed, and the boys were glaring at me.

"Hey, Guys!" I said, trying to play it cool. "How was your day?"

"Why didn't you come out with your class?" Mom asked.

"Because I stayed in the classroom and then fell asleep," I said matter of factly, hoping I could get away with it.

"Why did you stay in the room?" Mrs. Green asked, looking over her glasses at me.

"Well...um… you see…," I hesitated, still not wanting to say it.

"Mitchell," Mrs. Fields asked, "do you have something to tell your mother?"

"Yeah, um… I failed my classes."

"Why didn't you ask Dad or me for help?"

"I don't know. I guess I thought I could do it on my own."

"Well," Mom said, "I thought you fixed it since you didn't say anything." I could feel my eyes start to well up.

"It's going to be okay," Mrs. Fields said. "We have a plan."

"What is it?" I asked.

"Well, Mrs. Green and I talked at lunch today, and we decided that she will be helping you with your classes."

"How?"

"You will be coming to my classroom in the morning and read," Mrs. Green explained, "and when the kindergarten has left for the day, we will work on your other subjects."

"When would this start?" I asked excitedly.

"Monday," said Mrs. Green. "Don't go to the sixth-grade class. Just come down with Luke." I smiled because I knew that I would not have to be in a room with so many people who didn't like me.

Mom was not as excited about the idea. She knew for sure that this was the beginning of the end for my time at OLP. In her defense, up to that point, it was the right school for me. To this day, Mrs. Green is my favorite teacher, but the school was just not a good fit anymore. That night when everyone was asleep, Mom walked down the stairs, sat on the couch, and started crying. Looking for someone to confide in```1, she decided to text Robin. The texts went as follows:

Mom: Robin, are you still up?
Robin: Yes, are you okay?
Mom: No. Mitchell is failing his classes, and I don't think OLP is good for him anymore.
Robin: I think I might have a school for him.
Mom: Really? What's it called?
Robin: Haugland Learning Center, It's for people with autism.
Mom: I told you he has been in testing for autism.
He doesn't have it.
Robin: I think he does. I have had a few patients with it. It's not very prominent, but I think he does have it.
Mom: So, what do you think we should do?
Robin: Get him through the rest of the year, and you, Jerry, and I will do research. Then we will figure this out. I'm telling you, Sandra, everything is going to be okay.

CHAPTER 7: THE WILL EFFECT
12/25/2009-7/5/2010

On Christmas Day that year I woke up at Six a.m. I got out of bed and entered my parents' room to find that Ryan was already there. I greeted my parents and my brother with "Merry Christmas" and hugs. After a few minutes Mom and Dad told us to wake up Luke and Josh so we can pray the rosary, as we do every Christmas morning.

"...O Mother of the Word Incarnate, despise not my petitions, but in your mercy hear and answer me. Amen." When we finished praying the rosary, the boys and I ran down the stairs into the living room. The smell of plastic filled my nostrils, and the shiny, multi-colored wrapping paper was almost blinding. We collected the presents from under the tree and organized them by who they belonged to. Mom always wanted to get a video for every gift opened, so she made us take turns. This particular year Ryan was ready to start before the rest of us.

Everyone in my family, except myself, would open their presents from smallest to largest to prolong the experience. So, when he was ready, Mom turned on the camera, and Ryan reached for his tiniest gift.

"Oh!" Mom exclaimed. "Ryan, maybe you should wait to open that."

"Why?"

"Because I think I saw that Santa got the same thing for Mitchell."

"What?" I said. "I don't see one."

"I will help you find it," Dad said. "Ryan, open the next one, and on Mitchell's turn, you can open them together." Ryan did as he was told and reached for the second smallest gift. When the wrapping paper was removed, we saw an image of a green RC on the box. Right above the picture were the words, "The Frog." It was an appropriate name because the windows on it looked like eyes. Matched with the green color, it did look like a frog. A smile crept across his face, and he thanked "Santa." Luke went next, and by the time Josh went, I had found the box.

"Open on 'three.'" Mom said. "One, two, three." We pulled off the paper in a second flat. We both held in our hands a Tracfone.

"YESSS!" I screamed as I pulled it out of the box.

"Wow!" Ryan said.

"So, boys," Dad said, looking directly at me, so I knew he was not talking to Ryan, "Santa was nice enough to get you those. As long as you keep your grades up, you can keep them."

"Okay, Dad," I said, giving him a wink. "Can we set them up?"

"Let's just wait until we are done opening presents," Mom suggested. So, I waited, and waited, and waited. All of the other presents were cool, but all I wanted to do was play with my new phone. Just when I felt like I was about to explode, we finished opening all of the presents. As promised, we set up our phones right away.

"Hey, Ryan?" I asked when we had set them up. "What's your number?"

"Ummm… hold on a second," He looked at his phone and then said. "202-555-0130."

"Thank you," I said. "I'm going to send you a text." I wrote a message and hit send.

The rest of the school year went by in the blink of an eye. With the motivation of keeping my phone and the help of Mrs. Green, I managed to pass the sixth grade. The bullying didn't stop, so I was excited about the break. The summer was uneventful until July 5.

I know I touched on the Will effect before; his positive attitude makes people around him overexcited. What I did not say about it is what it could do for people like me. As a result of all the bullying I had been through at OLP I did not have high self-esteem. Fortunately, that was about change.

I stayed up late on the 4th, so I slept until about noon. I rolled out from the bottom bunk and stretched. I opened the door and called for Mom.

"She's not here," Luke squeaked from Mom and Dad's room. I entered and looked at him. He was lying on his stomach, in his pajamas, thumb in his mouth, watching a show on Nick Jr.

"Where is she?"

"At the studio with Daddy. They said they wanted to talk to you about something."

"What?"

"I don't know. They just said to call them when you got up."

"I'll go do that now." I re-entered my room and grabbed my phone. I noticed that Ryan had texted me. Our conversation went something like this:

Ryan: Hey, r u up yet?
Me: Yeah, u okay?
Ryan: Yes, I'm fine. Is Luke?
Me: Yes… dude, what's going on?
Ryan: Will and I r at the Duck Pond. We were playing with "The Frog," and it flipped over in the water. Could you come down and bring the string?
Me: On our way!!!

"Hey, Luke. Get dressed!" I called as I pulled the shirt over my head.

"Why?"

"Ry-Ry and Will need us. Hurry and meet me outside!" I ran down the stairs, and I dashed to a cabinet, right by the kitchen. I swung the cabinet-door open, a bit too dramatically, and I looked inside. On the top shelf, surrounded by markers and other arts and crafts materials, was a spool of white string covered in plastic wrap. "Bingo!" I said, grabbing it along with a pair of scissors. "COME ON, LUKE!" I called, sliding on my sandals.

"I CAN'T FIND PANTS!!!"

"WELL, LOOK HARDER!" I yelled, and I walked out the door. We had a huge back porch that Dad had made out of composite decking. Directly outside the door was a long brown picnic table and six wicker chairs. I sat at the head of the table and looked at the back yard.

A large brown garage was on the north side of the property. Directly behind the garage was a garden filled with a small apple tree, a blueberry bush, and many other plants that I could not name to save my life. About a foot behind that sat a rock formation that resembled a crescent moon. In the middle of the crescent was an old, rusty fire pit. A sea of ivy stretched from the south side of the half-moon to a fence that marked the Andersons' yard. The fence sagged in as the ivy climbed up and over. The fence ran the whole length of our backyard.

As I stood looking around, waiting for Luke, I heard loud voices coming over the fence. I jumped up, ready to tell whoever was talking to shut up. I ran to the fence and looked through a hole. On the back porch stood Arden with a red video camera; Lo-lo Anderson, a 6-year-old with hair that went all the way past her shoulders; and a tan girl from up the street named Shelby Jackson dancing around in front of the camera.

"So, they're hanging out with Shelby now? Great!" I said under my breath.

"Arden," Lo-lo asked, "are you sure we are doing it right? I mean, we don't have the song playing!"

"I promise we are doing it right." Arden replied, "just mouth the words, and I will add the music in editing." I wanted to yell at them, but as I was thinking of something to say, I heard the back door close, and Luke walked out. I knew that I could bug the girls whenever I wanted, but Ryan needed me right then. I ran back to the porch, grabbed the spool and scissors, and started running to the Duck Pond.

***

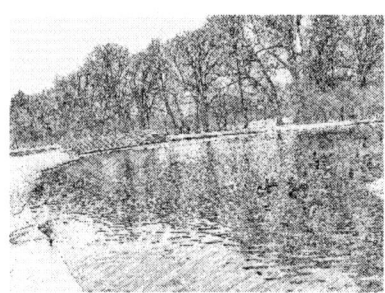

The Duck Pond was in the middle of a park, shaped like a figure eight. Across the middle of the eight was a gray wooden bridge. On the perimeter were a few benches, and about 150 feet away was a huge playground. When Luke and I finally made it, Ryan and Will were sitting on one of the benches on the left side of the pond.

"Hey!" Will said as he hopped up to meet us. "It's about time."

"Sorry," I said, "Luke couldn't find pants."

"Well," Will said, moving his blond curly hair out of his face, "you're here now! Are you ready, Luke?"

"Yes," Luke replied, still out of breath.

"I can't hear you!"

"YES."

"ONE MORE TIME!"

"YESSS!!!" Luke yelled, jumping up and down on the balls of his feet. As I watched Luke get more and more excited, I fell under the Will effect.

"Okay. Let's do this!" Will cheered.

"Where is it?" I asked.

"Over here," Ryan said, pointing to the middle of the left side of the pond.

"Ryan!" Will shouted, with his hand outstretched. "Branch!" Ryan grabbed a long-pointed tree-branch from the ground. He told me then to give him the spool and the scissors. He cut off some string, and he tied one end to the branch, and the other he tied into a loop. "Let's try this!" Will said as he swung the string towards the frog. He missed and tried again and again. After ten minutes, he got the string right on top of it, but the loop was too small.

"What if," Ryan suggested, "we poke it with the end of the branch?"

"Ah, that could work," Will replied, tentatively moving the branch towards its target.

"Come on," I whispered in anticipation.

"Almost got it," he said as he thrust it forward. He managed to move the toy, but the branch fell under the water and got stuck on something. After struggling for a few minutes, Ryan put his hand on Will's shoulder.

"It's okay," he said with a smile. "It will float to the edge at some point, and we will get it. Come on, let's go home. I will come and check tomorrow."

"Yeah, I guess," Will said, looking defeated.

I looked at Will in shock. I knew it was just a toy, and I understood that Ryan was trying to keep Will from feeling bad, but I couldn't believe that Will of all people was giving up. I was so gung-ho about this. I was not going to give up.

"Well, I have to go to the bathroom," I stated matter of factly.

"Can you wait?" Ryan asked.

"I mean there's a Porta John over by the playground. You guys go, and I will meet you at home."

"Okay," said Will. I started to walk to the playground, looking over my shoulder to see when they had left. When I could not see them anymore, I walked back to the pond's edge, and I took off my sandals. When I had aptly prepared myself, I jumped in.

The water jumped up on me only to splash away right after. It was warm, and an odor that I did not smell before I jumped assaulted my nose. I could feel that a net covered the entire bottom of the pond.

"Oh," I said. "That's how it got stuck." I looked at the branch as it peeked out of the waves I had made. As I watched, a Canadian goose landed to the right of the frog. I had seen videos of kids being attacked by geese, so I knew to steer clear. I trudged toward the branch as slowly as I could. When I got there, I wrapped my fingers around the top, and I pulled down. My plan was to break the branch, so if the goose attacked me, I could defend myself; unfortunately, things would not go according to plan.

The branch snapped and slipped beneath the water. I had not been ready to go under, and my mouth and eyes were open. Green water filled my mouth and burned my eyes. I stood up and coughed. As I rubbed my eyes, I heard an angry squawk, and wings started flapping. I removed my hands from my eyes and saw that part of the branch had flipped and hit the goose, and it was now heading right for me.

I looked around in a panic. I knew I couldn't get to the broken branch without getting even closer to my adversary. I noticed on my right was the bridge. I dove under the water and swam, escaping by the skin of my teeth. I hid under the bridge until the bird gave up. "Well, that was interesting," I said, excited to retrieve my prize.

CHAPTER 8: THE NEW SCHOOL

07/05/2010

"You got it?" Will screamed in disbelief when I got home.

"Yep!" I said proudly. "I had to outsmart a goose!"

"What?" the boys asked. I explained what had happened, and they couldn't believe it.

"Mitchell!" Mom yelled, running out the door. "Where have you been?"

"I got Ryan's toy out of the Duck Pond."

"Ah. No, wonder you smell! I told you to text me when you got up!"

"Oh yeah!" I exclaimed, remembering Luke passing on the message. "Sorry, I forgot. What did you want?"

"Go inside and take a quick shower. Dad will be home in ten minutes, and we are going to look at a new school." I looked at her, confused. "Just go. I'll explain when you get out." I obeyed and got in the shower. When I got out, my parents rushed me out the door and into our Honda minivan.

"So…" I stared after about 10 minutes of driving, "What's going on?"

"Well," Mom said delicately from the passenger seat, "you know how Robin is a nurse?"

"Yeah?"

"She works with lots of people, and you remind her of people who have something called autism."

"Au-ti-sm," I said slowly, "what is that?"

"It's a learning disability," Mom said.

"What does that mean?"

"All it means, Mitchell," Dad interjected, "is that you think differently than other people. It's why you're having so much trouble in school and why it's harder for you to make friends."

"Oh. Well, that makes sense," I said. "So, why are we going to a new school?"

"This is a school exclusively for kids with autism," Mom replied.

"Why are we going today?"

"Today is their ice cream social."

"When will we be there?"

"About five minutes." I watched the clock tick, and as time ran out, I became more and more excited. We finally parked, and I jumped out of the car. We walked into a building that looked like it had once been an office. A sea of children ranging all ages ran around laughing and screaming.

"Hello!" said a woman who approached us. "Welcome to Haugland Learning Center (HLC). I'm Kathy."

"I'm Jerry," Dad said, extending his hand. "This is my wife, Sandra, and this is our son Mitchell."

"Nice to meet you!" Kathy said to all of us. "Has he been diagnosed?"

"No, but our friend thinks he is on the spectrum," Mom replied.

"Will we get ice cream?" I asked.

"Yeah," Kathy said with a chuckle. "We will work our way to the cafeteria." And with that, we were off. As we walked, Kathy introduced us to teachers and staff and explained some of the protocols used in school. After about thirty minutes, we got to the lunchroom.

There were lunch tables set up along the back wall. Behind all the tables were adult volunteers serving ice cream. On the back wall, there was a long glass window and a door to its left. The door had a sign on it that said, "school store." I wanted the ice cream too much to care about what that meant. I ran ahead of the group and walked up to a table.

"Hi! What can I get you?" asked the woman behind the table.

"I'll have vanilla with fudge and sprinkles, please."

"Chocolate or rainbow sprinkles?"

"Rainbow."

As she got to work, I started jumping on the balls of my feet.

"You like ice cream?" the woman asked, seeing my excitement.

"Yeah," I said, looking right at the ice cream in anticipation. "My best friend and I--." I froze. Sam's face flashed before my eyes for just a second.

"Are you okay?" the woman asked, obviously concerned.

"Yes, ma'am, I am!" I lied. "Do you like ice cream?"

"Of course," she said. "Not as much as my son, but yes!"

"Who is your son?"

"His name is Zack," she said while handing me the ice cream. "He's in the game room playing Mario Kart."

"Wait. This place has a game room?"

"Yes, and they have all kinds of games and consoles!"

"Where is this game room?" I asked, a bit too enthusiastically.

She led me around a corner and into the game room. On the walls were images of cool video game characters. Three TVs were lined up against the wall, each running a different game. 15-20 kids were huddled around the screens. In the middle of one of the groups was a boy with short, blond hair, a round face, and green eyes.

"Zack!" the woman called. In response to her call, everyone turned to look at us. Now under normal circumstances, I would have felt uncomfortable with this many people looking at me. However, jumping into the pond prolonged the Will effect, so I felt confident.

"What?" Zack asked, irritably.

"This is..." she said, motioning to me. "I'm sorry, what's your name?"

"Mitchell."

"Thank you. This is Mitchell, and he would like to play with you guys. Is that okay?" The group all said it was okay, so I joined in. The whole time I was watching, I could not stop jumping around. I was so excited because, for the first time ever, a big group of people actually liked me.

"So," Zack asked after a couple of minutes, "why are you so happy?" I froze. I didn't want to say that I was happy to be included because I didn't want them to know I was usually an outsider.

"Well," I said, thinking on my toes, "I had an awesome day!"

"What happened?" Zack asked, and the whole group leaned in. I explained what had happened at the Duck Pond, and the kids went nuts! If I had told that to anyone at OLP, they would have given me some mean nickname, but these kids liked me! I knew if I kept doing crazy things, I would always be able to make friends at this school. Hearing the ruckus, Kathy ran in. She was followed closely by my parents.

"What's going on?" Kathy asked.

"Sorry," I said, running up to them. "Everyone liked my story. Mom, Dad, I'm never leaving this school!"

CHAPTER 9: THE FIRST BEHAVIOR

07/05/2010-08/19/2010

While Mom and Dad were excited about how much I like the school, they were still a little unsure about if I was autistic and if I could get in. Kathy reassured my parents by saying, "Oh, he's one of us!"

With our minds made up, we went to a doctor who worked for the school to confirm or deny Kathy's hunch. She told us that I have a mild form of autism called Asperger's syndrome. I was told that people who have Asperger's can become extraordinarily furious and are often socially awkward. They can have all-consuming obsessions with a particular topic, such as my love for *Blue's Clues* when I was a kid. The mind of an autistic person is wired differently than other people, so we have trouble learning by conventional means.

As we talked, I became more and more convinced that this woman had been following me all my life because she wasn't describing some disability. She was describing every single part of my personality. I became even more excited about the school because if one person who worked for the school could understand me like this, everyone probably would.

When the first day of school came around, I was actually excited for summer to end. I got up, got dressed, had breakfast, brushed my teeth, grabbed my backpack, and got into Mom's minivan.

"You ready?" Mom asked when she finally got into the car.

"Yes! Come on, let's go!" I exclaimed, and with that, we were off. Time seemed to slow down, and I became more and more excited.

"Have a nice day," Mom said when we got to the school. "Love you!"

"Love you too!" I said, jumping out of the car. I swung my backpack over my shoulder, closed the car door, and walked into the school. When I got into the school, I pulled out a paper schedule that Mom had printed off for me the night before. After a bit of exploring, I found my first class.

Six empty desks sat facing a whiteboard. In the bottom, the left-hand corner of the whiteboard, the word "marks" was underlined. In the middle, the name "Derek" was written. In the back of the room was the tallest person I had ever seen. His hair was red and curly. As I walked through the door, the man turned around.

"Well, hello there," he said with a smile. "I'm Derek. What's your name?"

"Hi, I'm Mitchell. Are you the teacher?"

"Yes, I am! Well, Mitch, you're the first person here. You get to choose the first seat." While I was slightly caught off guard by the nickname, he gave me, I was excited by it. It was like I was given a fresh identity, and I could be whoever I wanted to be.

I walked up to the front of the classroom and sat in the seat closest to the whiteboard. After about three minutes, another boy walked in the door. He was wearing a white shirt that read "I heart movies" on the front.

"Max!" Derek exclaimed when the boy walked in. The boy, Max, hugged Derek, and after a small conversation, he sat down at the desk next to mine.

"Hi!" I said, trying to start up a conversation.

"Hi!" he repeated.

"I'm Mitche-Mitch Ulibarri," I said.

"I'm Max O'Neil," he replied.

"So, what kind of movies do you like?" I asked.

"Mostly horror, but I watch a bunch of stuff."

"Oh, I've never seen a horror movie."

"You have not lived!" he exclaimed. "You need to come to my house, and we can have a marathon."

"Okay," I said. I felt conflicted. I knew I would hate a horror marathon, but this was the fastest friendship I had ever made in school. When all of the seats were filled up, Derek walked up to the front of the class.

"Good morning, everybody!" he said, quieting the classroom. "As some of you may have noticed, we have a new student with us today." I waved to the class and introduced myself. "It's nice to have you, Mitch." After Derek had Max explain how class is worked at Haugland, he started teaching.

At the end of class, Max and I exchanged numbers, and I walked to my next class. When I walked in the door, I saw three people talking. The first person was Zack. The second person was another boy and the third was a girl. She was beautiful. Her eyes were like emeralds, and her hair was like gold. Her voice was soft, and her smile was kind.

"Well, well, well," said Zack when he saw me. "If it isn't pond boy!"

"Pond boy!" I exclaimed. "Is that really the nickname you're going with?"

"Why would you call him that?" asked the boy. Zack began to tell the story (with incredible accuracy, I might add) to his friends.

"Oh my gosh!" the girl said when Zack was done. "You're awesome! What's your name?"

"Mitch Ulibarri."

"I'm Caroline Knight, and that's my former best friend, Jake Campbell," she said, pointing to the boy.

"What do you mean 'former'?" Jake asked.

"Well," Caroline said while putting her arm on my shoulder. "You, sir, have officially been replaced." My face felt like it had caught fire because I was blushing so hard.

"Wow," said Jake sarcastically. "Obviously, I'm not that important to you!"

"Yes, Jake," she replied. "I've been waiting for the last two years to get rid of you." She joked. We talked until class started.

"Say," Caroline said to me as we got to our seats, "would you like to come to eat lunch with us?" I was shocked because she had to be the prettiest girl in the school, and she was asking me, the new kid, to sit with her group.

"Me?" I asked. "You want me to sit at lunch with you and your friends?"

"Yeah, sure!" she said. "Why not? You seem cool."

"Okay," I said, "I'll meet you in the lunchroom then!"

***

I walked into lunch and looked for my newfound friends. The lunchroom was full, so I was lost until I saw Zack waving at me from the back. There were four chairs at the table. Caroline and Zack were sitting with their backs to the wall while Jake sat across from Caroline. I took the only seat left, which was right next to Jake, and we all started talking. They asked me how I found HLC, who I hung out with before, and I answered all of their questions. Everything was normal and calm until about halfway through lunch.

All of a sudden, a blood-curdling scream erupted from directly behind me. It was the kind of scream you only hear in nightmares or in horror movies. The sound rushed through my body and turned my bones to jelly. I slowly turned around to see who had emitted the sound.

There were two boys behind me. One of them had his back to me. He was tiny, and he was bracing himself. In comparison the other boy who had let out the scream was monstrous. He kept screaming, and he charged and attempted to attack the smaller kid.

A teacher on the other side of the room ran to the little kid's defense, pulled out a camo walkie-talkie and said, "Behavior support to the lunchroom. Behavior support to the lunchroom." In response to the teacher's actions the kid who had been yelling, turned his attention to the teacher.

"Just ignore it, everybody!" The teacher said to the room as he blocked the kid's strikes. Everyone just kept talking like nothing was happening.

"What the heck is going on?" I asked my table.

"He's having a behavior!" everyone said in unison.

"Well, obviously!" I exclaimed. "I mean, why is everybody acting like this is normal?"

"Because it is!" Zack said.

"Here they come," said Jake. I looked up just as three men ran to help. They came from behind the boy, and all three of them assisted the teacher in getting him under control. This took a while and the boy would not stop screaming. All I could do was watch in awe and confusion.

"Just ignore it," Caroline said, reaching across the table to grab my hand. I pulled away. How could anyone ignore this? The boy was cursing at the teachers and saying terrible things about the little boy. In the end the event resolved itself and no one was injured. While I loved Haugland I did hate it when the students got upset. I wanted to help them feel better and I hoped I would never have to see any of my friends go through that.

CHAPTER 10: THE DOCTOR

09/15/2010

A month passed, and everything was relatively "normal." I embraced my weirdness and the weirdness of my new school. The weirder I got, the more friends I made, and the higher my self-esteem became. I was way happier than I had been in years, and it was about to get even better.

In the middle of September was when *it* happened. The day started out like any other morning, for the most part. I got ready a lot faster than usual because I could not wait to talk to Max. Greg had just shown me the original *Iron Man*, and I knew Max would be excited when I told him. I arrived at school 20 minutes early and started to look for Max, but what I found made all of my excitement dwindle.

I found Max in the hallway outside of Derek's classroom, but he was not alone. Aidan, another student from Derek's class, stood right in front of Max. Aidan's finger was in Max's face, and about three or four kids were watching.

"Well, go on!" Aidan shouted, stepping closer and closer to Max. "What are you looking at?"

"I... I... I…" Max said.

"You... You... You what?" he mocked. Max hung his head and tried to avoid eye contact. I threw off my backpack and started to run in hopes that I could get Max out of the situation. "I guess I shouldn't expect much of a response from a r***rd like--"

"HEY!" I exclaimed, stepping between them. "Don't call him that ever!"

"Why not? He is!"

"SHUT UP!" Max yelled from behind me. Aidan's eyes widened in fear, so I knew that Max was about to attack. I began to panic. All I could think about was the lunchroom incident and every incident I had seen after. Every time was the same as the first: a kid would get upset and would not stop screaming until behavior support arrived. Most of the time even then they would still be upset for a while. I didn't want to see Max upset or Aidan get hurt so I tried to protect him.

I grabbed Aidan by his right shoulder and pushed him out of the way. He lost his balance and fell at the feet of the bystanders. I turned on my heel and faced Max, who was charging right at Aidan. I stood in his way and put an end to his sudden attack.

"GET OUT OF MY WAY!" he yelled.

"No," I said calmly.

"He called me a r***rd!"

"I know, and there is _no excuse_ for him to say that, but--." Before I could finish my sentence, I was face down on the ground. Confused, I rolled over onto my back. Aidan stood over me with a cruel smile. He fell on top of me, landing his knee on my chest. All of the air was forced out of my body.

"You should have stayed out of this," he said over-dramatically. Aidan started hitting and scratching my face and neck. Time slowed down and seemingly stopped. I could hear the bystanders screaming, so I knew a teacher would be coming soon. I blocked and tried to fight back as much as I could but so much was happening, I didn't know what to do.

Out of the corner of my eye, I saw Caroline running towards us. She got right next to us, brought her leg up, and kicked Aidan in the side. He let out a gasp and stopped his attack. I put my hands on his chest and pushed him off. He landed and looked at Caroline so intently that I thought he was drilling a hole in her head with his eyes. I pulled myself up and stood next to her.

"Good...morning!" I said between gasps. "What a beautiful day!"

"Shut up!" Caroline replied.

"You little b****!" Aidan screamed, lunging at Caroline. Right before he could reach her, Derek appeared and restrained Aidan. As he was brought to the ground, Aidan's eyes never left Caroline and me. "I hate you!!!" he screamed. "When I get out of this, I swear, I'm gonna beat the living sh** out of you!!! I'm going to make both of you pay!!!!"

"No, you're not," Derek said firmly. "You will apologize to them." Derek looked at me and continued. "Mitch, go to the bathroom and clean up."

"What?" I asked.

"You're bleeding," Caroline explained. I touched my neck, and sure enough, my hand came back red. I hadn't even noticed!

"Just wash it off," Derek said. "I have band-aids on my desk."

"You deserve it!" Aidan sneered. "That's what you get for defending Max!"

"Shut up!!!" Max yelled. When I saw that Max was upset, my gut was to try and make him feel better.

"Max," I said, putting my hand on his shoulder, "please stop."

"No!" he repeated, putting his foot down instead of kicking.

"Why not?" I asked.

"Because," he said while glaring at me, "I just looked at him and he got in my face! Then he called me a r***rd, choked you, and called Caroline a b****! He deserves this!"

"Max, I understand, trust me. There are these girls that I used to be friends with. They made my brother cry, and I attack them all the time because they deserve it, but this is different."

"How?"

"Well, are you a r***rd?"

"No!"

"Is Caroline a... um, a... you know?"

"No."

"If you just looked at him and he got mad at you, then who has the problem?"

"Him."

"Then let's let Derek and the behavior support handle this. Okay?"

"Okay," he said, starting to walk away from Aidan. "Let's go to class."

"I will meet you there," I said. "Caroline, can you wait in the classroom with him?" Caroline's eyes widened, her mouth was hung open, and she was looking right at me. For a second, I thought she was looking at something right behind me. I turned, and nobody was there. "Caroline?"

"Huh… yeah?"

"Can you wait with him in Derek's classroom? I'm gonna clean up."

"Of course," she said as she and Max walked away. When I got to the classroom, Max and Caroline looked up at me and were both smiling.

"What?" I asked.

"Mitch," Caroline said, "that was amazing!"

"Really?" I asked.

"Yeah, man," Max said, "I've never been calmed down that fast in my entire life!"

"It was like," Caroline continued, "you were a psychiatrist, and you knew what he was thinking."

"Well, I didn't know what to do, but no 'thanks' required," I said, taking a bow. "Dr. John Mitchell Ulibarri, at your service."

"Dr. Mitch!" Max exclaimed. Caroline and I looked at Max.

"Dr. Mitch," I said. "I like it!"

CHAPTER 11: THE MOVIE PART 1
09/15/2010-11/19/2010

At lunch that day, Caroline gathered a group of kids around herself and I. She told the story to the group, and when she had finished, they all looked at me like I was a celebrity.

My name had kind of gotten around before this point because of the Duck Pond incident, but after a week, I was the most popular person in school. All of a sudden, I had more friends than I knew what to do with. Life was almost perfect; keyword: *almost*.

As you, the reader, know, I grew up in an intimate friendship with the Anderson girls. Now I had more friends than I could count. However, because I had so many friends, the friendships felt reasonably empty.

The Thursday before Thanksgiving, Max asked me if I wanted to hang out the next day. So, the next day I left school with him. We walked up to his red truck.

"I'll sit in the back with you," Max said.

"Works for me," I said.

"Hi, Mom!" he said.

"Hey, Max!" his mom replied. "How was your day?"

"It was good!"

"That's great!" She looked at me. "You must be 'Dr. Mitch.'"

"At your service," I said, extending my hand while bowing.

"Wow!" she exclaimed with a chuckle. "You weren't kidding. Max, he is eccentric."

"I told you!"

"Yeah," I said, "it's a fairly new thing."

"Well, I think it's awesome, and I know Max thinks the same."

"Thank you," I replied happily.

"You're welcome!" she replied as we drove off. "So, any plans for Thanksgiving?"

"My grandpa and my aunt always come up from Florida, and my mom's family comes over. What are you guys doing?"

"We just have our family over," Max said as he pulled out an iPad. He went to the camera app and started to scroll. He got to a photo and stopped. The photo was of him and his family. He pointed to every member and told me who they were.

***

We got to his house half an hour later. Right inside the door was a wooden staircase. As soon as we walked in, two tiny dogs bolted down the stairs and jumped up at us, begging us to pet them.

"Calm down, guys!" Max's mom said. "We have company!"

"Sorry, Mitch!" Max said.

"No, it's fine. I don't mind," I said while petting the one that was in front of me.

"So, what do you want to do?" Max asked.

"I don't know," I said, shrugging. "It's your house. What do you usually do?"

"Watch movies."

"That's fine."

"Okay, cool!" he said. "Come with me."

I followed Max and the dogs up the stairs. At the top of the stairs was a blue carpeted hallway. Max made a right turn towards a door at the end of the hall. The door was closed, and on it was a paper sign that said, "Max's Cinema." The room had two humongous bookshelves on the back wall. The bookshelves held hundreds if not thousands of movies on them. Movie posters plastered the walls, and a TV sat on a desk at the end of his bed.

"Wow!" I exclaimed.

"What do you think?" Max asked, outstretching his arms and raising them to his shoulders.

"Wow," I repeated. "I don't think I've ever seen this many movies in one place."

"Thank you," he said. "What do you want to watch?"

"What do you recommend?"

"Umm," he said, hesitating, "*Saw* is pretty good."

"Okay, let's do it," I said. Now, I grew up pretty sheltered. I'd never seen a horror movie; I didn't even know what *Saw* was. By the two-minute mark, I was about ready to crap my pants. Luckily, I was about to be saved. There was a knock at the door 15 minutes into the movie.

"Max?" a girl said from the other side of the door.

"Yes?" Max responded.

"Can I come in?"

"Sure!" The door opened as she strutted in. I recognized the girl from the picture Max had shown me. It was Sally, his sister.

"Whatcha' doing?" Sally asked.

"Just watching a movie with Mitch."

"Ah, of course. Hi Mitch!" she said, turning to me. "Hi," I said sheepishly.

"Are you okay?" Max asked.

"Yes," I lied.

"Are you scared?" Sally mouthed to me, raising her eyebrows. I nodded in reply. "Hey, Max, let's do something else."

"Why?"

"Umm…" Sally said, looking at me and then back at Max, "it's such a nice day out. You don't want to waste it, do you?"

"What would we do?" Sally sat down on Max's bed right next to him, and she smiled. "What?"

"What's better than watching a movie?" she asked, excitedly.

"Making a movie!" Max said, producing the same excitement. "I'm going to get my camera. You guys meet me downstairs!" I watched Max run out of his room.

"Thanks," I said to Sally, when he was out of earshot, "I've seen things no man should see!"

"No problem," she said, stifling a laugh. "Go on. I will meet you guys after I put the movie away."

For the next hour and a half, Max, Sally, and I ran around the backyard filming our very own movie. I have been thinking about it for weeks on end, and for the life of me, I can't remember what the movie was about. What I can remember is how fun it was. When we were done, Max, Sally, and I edited it, and we watched it on his mom's laptop. As soon as we finished watching it, all I wanted to do was make another one.

CHAPTER 12: THE MOVIE PART 2
11/24/2010-01/05/2011

The following Wednesday morning, I woke up to voices coming from downstairs. I sat up, hitting my head on the top bunk. As I rubbed the bump on my head, I remembered that Mom had gone to the airport the night before to pick up my aunt and grandpa.

I dashed down the stairs and slid into the kitchen. Ryan was sitting at the table with them. My grandpa had tan skin, gray curly hair, and stubble on his face. He sat at his MacBook, and he had a coffee mug in his hand. My aunt Eva had shiny, black hair and brown eyes.

"Pop-Pop! Eva!" I exclaimed.

"Hi, Mitchell!" Pop-Pop said, jumping up to hug me.

"Pop-Pop, any good stories?" I asked after I hugged Eva and him.

When he finished telling us about some shenanigan he got into recently, Ryan and I could not stop laughing. I started to stagger forward as I laughed, and I got right in front of the laptop. Facebook was pulled up on the screen.

"What's that?" I asked.

"Facebook," Pop-Pop said.

"What does that mean?"

"It's social media," Eva said.

"I'm sorry?" I said, still incredibly confused. Pop-Pop then demonstrated how it worked. "Ah! Do you think I could get one?" That was how I was introduced to social media. By the end of the day, I had become friends with about 15 people, one of them being Greg.

The next day, Mom's side of the family came for Thanksgiving as they do every year. Aunt Melissa and Uncle Andy brought their four kids, and Uncle Bob came with his future wife, Erin. Aunt Cindy arrived with her husband, Joey, and Nimba, and Jack (Papa) brought Shana's daughter Lexi.

After dinner, Joey started to play Dad's old guitar. The other kids and I saw him begin to play. We stopped what we were doing and sat down to watch him. About halfway through his first song, I looked over to my left. The other kids were sitting in a little group with looks of pure admiration on all of their faces. I stood up and ran to Mom.

"Hey, Mom!" I said when I found her talking to Aunt Melissa and Aunt Cyndi.

"What?" she asked suspiciously.

"Umm… can I have your phone?"

"Why?"

"I want to take a video."

"Again?"

"Yes!"

"What's going on?" Aunt Melissa asked.

"Last week, Mitchell and his friend made a movie, and since then, he has not wanted to stop taking videos on my phone," Mom explained.

"85 so far!" I exclaimed proudly.

"Really?" Aunt Cyndi asked, matching my enthusiasm.

"Yup! I just wish I could make more movies."

"Why can't you?" my aunts asked in unison.

"Cuz, I don't know who would want to."

"Well, how do you know?" Aunt Melissa asked.

"The boys have made it clear that they don't want to, and people at school probably wouldn't want to."

"Have you asked?"

"No. Max is the only person who seems interested in that kind of stuff."

"You should at least ask," Aunt Cyndi said. "You might be surprised."

"Okay," I said in response

When Thanksgiving Break ended, I told Caroline and the gang about my new obsession. To my surprise, they were all in. My aunts were right. "That's such a good idea, Mitch," Caroline said, putting her arms around me. "We should get like ten more people!"

"Thanks," I said blushing. "We only need nine because Max will probably join us."

"Okay, nine," she said, winking at me. Within two weeks, we got all of the people we needed. We all exchanged numbers and started making plans to meet. The first time we tried to hang out, Max forgot that we were meeting, so we did not have a camera. The next time, a few of us got sick, so we could not film everything we had planned. After that, everyone kind of gave up.

A couple of days before Christmas, every year, Mom's side of the family gets together to make Grandma Opper's homemade cut-out Christmas cookies. At some point during the process that year, Aunt Cyndi remembered what we had talked about at Thanksgiving about my desire to make movies. I told her what had happened and how it all ended up not working out. After she thought for a second, she said, "You know, if all else fails, you always have those girls."

"What girls?" I asked.

"The Andersons."

"Ummm…. no!"

"Why not?"

"Because they're mean!"

"You guys were so close. What happened? You've never talked about what happened."

"They changed."

"Did they, or did you?" Aunt Cyndi asked, looking deep inside me. I didn't respond.

"Look, who cares what happened. I think it's time to put it behind you." I did not care about putting it behind me. What I did care about was what I wanted to do right then, and the girls did offer something. I remembered that Arden had been making a video with Lo-lo and Shelby the summer before.

"Maybe you're right," I said, keeping my scheme from her.

"I always am!" she replied.

I spent the next two weeks figuring out how to ask them. I knew that because of my history with the girls, they would not be receptive to my proposal, so I came up with an ingenious lie to get them to do it. By the first few days of 2011, I was ready to ask. Soon after I had finished planning, I looked out the window and froze.

***

"Come with us," Arden said, walking towards the house.

"You're on thin ice, Mr.!" August said as we walked to their side door. My hands were shaking, and I couldn't believe that this plan had a slight chance of working. Arden opened the side door, and we walked in.

"WHAT IS *HE* DOING IN MY HOUSE!?" Aspen yelled.

"Apparently," August said sarcastically, "he has a school project he needs our help with."

"WHY WOULD WE HELP YOU? WE CAN'T EVEN TRUST YOU!"

"Apparently he can 'earn our trust.'"

"PFFF, YEAH, RIGHT!"

"Come on, guys!" Arden interrupted. "Give him a chance. Mitchell, what's this movie project."

"First off, it's Mitch now."

"We're not calling you Mitch," August interrupted.

"Well, it's my name!" I continued. "Second, I'm sorry about everything, and I can earn your trust. Third, there's this kid in my class, and he loves movies. He didn't have a behavior for a whole month, so the teacher let him make his own lesson. By the beginning of March, I need to have a movie done for credit because that is part of his lesson."

"Are you sure?" Arden asked.

"Yes."

"What's your friend's name?" August asked.

"Max."

"Teacher's name?" Arden asked once again.

"Derek."

"Are you sure this is not for Facebook?" Aspen asked.

"How do you know I have a Facebook?"

"Melody said you added Greg."

"Ah. No, it's not for Facebook."

"Okay, we will need to talk about this in private," August said.

"So, when do I come back?" I asked.

"Do you have a phone?" Arden asked.

"Yes."

"Here," she said, giving me her flip phone. "Put in your number, and I will call you." I did as I was told and handed her phone back to her.

"There you go," I said. "Thanks, guys. I really appreciate--"

"GO!" Aspen shouted, and so I ran out of the house.

Season 2: THE LIE

CHAPTER 13: THE ADVENTURE BEGINS

01/05/2011-01/08/2011

As I was leaving the Andersons' house, Rich, Lo-lo, and Shelby headed back from a walk with the Andersons' golden retriever, Maggie. When they saw me coming out of the house, they turned to stone.

"Hey, guys!" I said, walking up to them with confidence.

"Hello, Mitchell," Rich said. "What's going on?"

"Well, I need help from the girls! Go inside, they will explain it."

***

That day was a Wednesday. I could not stop looking at my phone throughout the following two days in hopes that Arden would call. The next Saturday, I woke up to the vibration of my phone.

"Hello?" I said, groggily.

"Hey, Mitchie!" Arden screamed.

"My gosh! It's too early for screaming, and my name is Mitch, not Mitchie!"

"Umm it's 1:30! Are you just getting up, Mitchie?"

"No--"

"Yes, you are!" the other girls said in the background.

"Fine!" I said.

"Are you gonna come over?" Arden asked.

"Right now? I have to get dressed and eat. Maybe in an hour?"

"What? An hour? You should come over now!"

"We have food here!" Lo-lo said.

"Yeah!" Arden continued. "Come on, Mitchie, please come over!"

"Yeah, come over!" the other girls chimed in.

"Okay, fine. On my way."

There's a saying about Ohio: "If you don't like the weather, wait 10 minutes." In other words, Ohio weather is bipolar. On that Saturday, frost and ice from the past few days had melted. As a result of the weather, Greg, Melody, and their dad were in the front yard.

"Hey, Mitchell!" Mr. Parker said when he saw me. Upon hearing my name, the kids both looked up. Greg smiled, and Melody gave me the death glare.

"What's going on?" Greg asked me.

"I'm going to the Andersons' house," I replied with confidence.

"Wait, what?" Greg asked. "Why?"

"We're friends now!"

"Yeah, right," Melody said with a chuckle.

"Okay," I said, "don't believe me, but I have to go." Greg and Melody looked at each other in confusion as I walked off. By the time I got to the Andersons' driveway, Melody had caught up to me. She walked next to me as I started up the driveway.

"What are you up to?" she asked.

"I need help with a project for school, and I think it's time we bury the hatchet." Melody lifted her eyebrows in suspicion. I knew that she could tell I was lying, so I knew that I had to look confident. I stood tall, and I tried to keep a straight face. She almost looked at me long enough for me to crack. Almost.

"Can I help?"

"Yeah, I'm sure we could find something for you to do."

"We already do!" shouted Arden from a window in the kitchen. We both jumped out of our skins.

"Why were you just standing there?" Melody asked.

"Just waiting to scare Mitchie!" Arden said between laughing fits.

"It's Mitch!"

"So, what do you have for me?" asked Melody, ignoring me. Arden beckoned us in the house. As we walked up the side door stairs, I saw Greg standing at the end of the driveway with his mouth wide open. We walked into the house, and Arden sat us around the kitchen table. The other three girls and Shelby were already there.

"So, what do you guys have in mind?" I asked, taking a chair.

"It's called *Miracle Child*," August said, pulling out a piece of paper and sliding it across the table. I picked up the paper and started to read:

Miracle Child

A couple (played by August and Arden) get engaged. A few years later, the husband gets a promotion. In celebration, the couple decides to take their new baby on vacation. The plane mysteriously crashes, and the only survivor is the baby.

A week later, a couple (played by Melody and Mitchie) go to an orphanage to adopt a baby. They recognize the "Miracle Child" from the news. They choose the miracle child and rename her Jessica. A year later, they had a son named Andrew. Young Jess and Andrew (played by Shelby and Luke) are raised by the couple until they are nine and ten when the couple passes away.

Jess and Andrew (now played by Aspen and Mitchie) are sent back to the orphanage. Jess has a dream about the crash, and she knows who is responsible. She tells Andrew everything, and they leave the orphanage on foot to find him. Andrew dies during the search for the culprit, and Jess returns to the orphanage.

As a result of the missing kids, the orphanage has to be shut down when Jess returns. She stays in the orphanage the last few nights that it is opened. She goes back to her old room, which is now a guy's (played by August) room. The two fall in love, grow up and get married. Together the new couple reopen the orphanage where they once fell in love.

"What do you think?" Arden asked when I looked up.

"You killed me off?"

"Yes," Aspen said.

"In my own movie!"

"I mean, I'm okay with it!" August said with a grin. Everyone busted out laughing.

"Har, har, har," I said. "But in all seriousness, it is terrific!"

"Great! Let's get started!" Arden said.

CHAPTER 14: THE SISTERHOOD

01/08/2011

While we filmed that Saturday, I realized how this group was structured. August kept telling people what she thought looked best, and everyone listened to her. In other words, August was the team leader. August and Arden seemed to have a symbiotic relationship. As a result, Arden was August's right-hand woman, but she had a more important job. She was the most compassionate member of the group. If a fight broke out or looked like one was about to happen, Arden would be the peacekeeper. Aspen was short-tempered. She always made sure that she was involved in the other girls' conversations or decisions. As a result, she was at the center of the group. Lo-lo was the group's gofer. If anyone asked for anything, she would get it. I was able to figure out everyone's role in the group within an hour. Well, everyone except Shelby. She was just kind of there.

I found Shelby extremely annoying. The reason was that when Shelby was about four years old, her best friend was the boy who lived next door to her. Shelby's parents would often take Shelby, her brother James, and the next-door neighbor boy down to the circle. When I would spot them outside, I genuinely didn't mind Shelby. I thought she was a cute kid but there was still a problem. Around the same time that I would see Shelby and her friend playing, the Andersons and I had started fighting. The following year, Shelby's friend moved away. To replace her old friend, Shelby began hanging out with Lo-lo.

The situation was a problem because of the bullying at OLP, and the fact that I was very lonely because the Andersons had stopped hanging out with me. As a result, I became very jealous of Shelby. The girls were *my* friends, and Shelby had no right to them.

Because of my issues with her, I noticed everything she did wrong. The whole time we were recording, she was sassing everybody. Any task we asked of her, she would scoff and roll her eyes. When Shelby *finally* left at about 9:00 P.M., I took Arden aside.

"Why do you guys put up with her?"

"With who? Oh, Shelby?"

"Yeah."

"She is Arlo's friend."

"I know, but she's so annoying. Why don't you make her go away when she acts like that?"

"We aren't that great at making friends. We want to hold on to as many as we can."

"I know the feeling… but come on, Shelby?"

"What do you think we were thinking the other day when you asked us to help you with this movie?"

"Touché."

"Look," Arden said, "try to tolerate her. She may be annoying, but if you get to know her, she's super awesome!"

"Okay, fine," I said, slightly disgruntled. I put on my shoes and started to walk out the door.

"Mitchie," Arden said, "Welcome to the sisterhood." I smiled and closed the door behind me.

CHAPTER 15: THE FOREST WITCH

01/13/2011

The next Thursday, I walked into the lunchroom before Caroline and the others. I found a table and sat down. Just as Caroline and Jake walked in, I waved at them. Caroline walked towards me while Jake ran the other way.

"What's with him?" I asked.

"He forgot his lunch box," she said. "So, I have a question for you." She started talking in a hushed tone that I had never heard her use.

"What is it?" I asked, putting my hands on the table and leaning in to hear.

"There's this boy," she started, putting her hands over mine. "I like him, and I think he likes me. He's awkward, so I don't think he is going to ask me out. What should I do?" My heart started pounding, and I felt a smile creep onto my face. "What?" she asked.

"I think I know who you are talking about."

"Oh, you do? So, what do you think?"

"I think you're right. *He* is way too awkward to ask you out. I think you should ask him."

"Okay, I will." I looked into her deep green eyes, waiting for her to ask.

"Well?"

"Well, what?"

"Ask!" I replied, just as she turned around and saw Jake.

"Oh, cool! Thanks, Mitch!" she said, standing up. She ran to him, and they talked for a second. Suddenly Jake put his hand behind her head and kissed her.

"No problem," I whispered.

***

When I got home that day, I went to work on *Miracle Child* at the Andersons' house to keep my mind off Caroline. When I knocked on the door, a girl I had never seen before opened it. She had blue eyes; curly, orange hair; and a look of confidence across her face.

"Hello, Mitchie!" she said with a grin.

"Who are you and how do you know me?" I asked.

"I know everything," she said creepily. My eyes widened, and my mouth dropped. August, Arden, Aspen, and Lo-lo popped out from behind the counter. They were all laughing hysterically. The new girl introduced herself. "I'm Arden's best friend, Tina!"

We talked for a while until I asked what we were going to do. Tina looked back at the Anderson girls, and they all looked at me and smiled. Their eyes raised as if implying that they had a few ideas. Within ten minutes, we were walking down towards the Duck Pond. Since it was early January, it was tremendously cold outside, but there wasn't any snow. I kept asking what we were doing, which caused them to giggle every time. We stopped on the bridge of the Duck Pond.

"It's time," August said, looking at Lo-lo. Lo-lo, in response, reached into her back pocket and pulled out a bandana.

73

"We can't show you where we're going."

"Oh, come on!" I exclaimed. "Why?"

"It's for your safety," Tina said nonchalantly. I looked around skeptically.

"You can't be serious!" I said.

"Serious as a heart attack!" Aspen retorted. I decided to play along as I wanted to get my mind off Caroline and because there was nothing better to do. August took the bandana from Lo-lo and placed it over my eyes.

I can't tell you exactly what happened in the next 10-15 minutes, but someone took my hand and started walking. Eventually, the ground became uneven, and I could hear a river off in the distance.

"Okay," Tina said, "wait right there." I thought she was saying stay in the general area, but she meant, "don't move at all, or you're going to hurt yourself!" I took a step forward only to walk directly into something hard.

"Ouch!" I exclaimed, removing the blindfold. Directly in front of me was a huge tree. I looked around and realized I was in a forest. A light frost covered the leaves that were on the ground. I rubbed my head, and everyone started laughing.

"I told you!" Tina yelled.

"Yeah, yeah, yeah," I said bitterly. "So, why are we down here?"

"Theodora's treasure," the girls said in unison.

"What?"

"Just follow us," August said.

I followed the girls down a small path that led to a clearing. Upon entering the clearing, I saw the river.

Right in the middle of the river was a rock formation that the water flowed over.

"Who is Theodora, and what is this treasure?" I asked.

The Anderson girls all looked at Tina. She took a deep breath and explained: "About 100 years ago, a girl named Theodora was born. She was the second born child. She and her older sister would often play in this very river, but there was something odd about Theodora. Ever since she was a little girl, she could make things happen. If she wanted to fly, she could fly. If she wanted to be somewhere, she was. If she wanted someone to get hurt, she would hurt them. One day, Theodora got in a fight with her sister. The next day her sister was found dead. Her parents tried to turn Theodora in for murdering their eldest daughter, but she used her powers and created this forest."

"Why are we here?" I asked, rolling my eyes.

"Last summer I came down here by myself and Theodora appeared. She cast a spell on me. She tethered me to a magical rock, and as long as she had that stone, I have to do what she wants," Tina replied.

I didn't believe a word she said, but I was bored and still didn't want to think about Caroline. So, I asked Tina what I had to do.

"It's a red rock, about the size of my palm," August explained, "and it's right in the river."

"If we take it out of the forest," Aspen expanded the obviously fake story, "the magic will be drained from it, and Tina will be free."

I walked to the river, and I could see the red rock was at the bottom, a few feet away from the rock formation. It was a little way in, so I would definitely have to get into the water. As I continued to look into the water, the wind started picking up.

"She's getting angry!" Tina yelled. "Hurry!"

I jumped in without hesitation. I screamed on impact due to the freezing water. The gang cheered me on as I slowly but surely inched my way towards the red rock. When I got right above the rock, I reached my hand in and grabbed it.

As I made it out of the creek, everyone cheered around me. They kept telling me Theodora was coming and that we had to run. I was shocked, and I couldn't think straight. Why were they making such a big deal out of this? It's just a game--and a bizarre one at that. But I think the reason I was so shocked was that even though I was cold and miserable, I was having fun with the Anderson girls.

We made it out of the forest and ran home. When we got back, I ran into my house to get some new clothes and then returned to their house. Tina's mom had arrived, and after five minutes of conversation, Tina and her mom drove home.

"So, what are we doing now?" I asked the girls.

"We can record until it's time for dinner!" Arden said. We started recording until Rich came home. The moment he walked in the door; the smell of pizza filled the house.

"Daddy!" the girls yelled, running to meet him at the door. I followed them. Once I confirmed that the smell was indeed pizza, I decided to let myself out the back.

"Hey, Mitchell!" Rich exclaimed. "Where are you going?"

I stopped and turned to look at him. "I'm going home."

"You know you can stay for dinner if you want." I smiled and laughed.

"Well," I replied, "I should probably get home. I don't want to impose--" Rich was about to tell me to have a good night when I raised my hands dramatically and continued. "but if you insist, I mean, I guess I can stay for free food."

"Well, okay then!" Rich said with a chuckle. "Come on, guys. Let's set the table and eat!"

CHAPTER 16: THE EXTERMINATOR
01/13/2011

As dinner went on, we got on the topic of "weirdest things that have happened to us." We went around the table and told our stories. When it was my turn, I told the story of when I jumped into the Duck Pond in excruciating detail. They all thought the story was hilarious. Aspen's story followed mine.

"Okay," she said, "but after this, I have to be excused because I have to go do homework."

"That's fine," Rich said. "Go ahead."

Aspen smiled, took a bite of pizza, and started the story. It went something like this: Aspen played lacrosse, and she was an aggressive player. Aspen played a game the season before when a girl on the other team was about to score. Aspen was the last line of defense before the goalie. Aspen charged the girl. The girl was caught entirely off guard, and Aspen took a chance and stole the ball from the girl.

Aspen dashed all the way down the field, shot the ball into the goal, and dramatically posed, holding her lacrosse stick above her head. For no reason at all, one of her teammates yelled, "Exterminator!" Aspen understood the teammate was excited and showing her support but still, a random thing to yell.

After the story was done, Aspen did as she said she would and left to do her homework. Soon after, everyone else got up from the table and threw the paper plates away.

August, Arden, and Lo-lo went to the sunroom to play with Maggie. I knew I had to go home soon because I hadn't told my family I was staying for dinner. While I was in the kitchen putting my shoes on, Barbara, Rich, and I started a conversation. We hadn't even been talking for a minute when Maggie began to bark.

"Oh my gosh!" August yelled.

"Ewwww!" Arden cried.

"Mommy!" Lo-lo called.

Without hesitation, Barbara and Rich ran into the sunroom with me close behind. A shrew was scurrying around the sunroom. Maggie was chasing it and trying to catch it. As soon as we entered the sunroom, the girls ran to us and started freaking out.

Barbara ran into the sunroom and retrieved Maggie because she didn't want Maggie to kill it and get blood everywhere. Rich just couldn't stop laughing.

"Mitchie, do something!" August ordered.

"What do you want me to do?"

"I don't know! Dad's not doing anything cuz he thinks this is hilarious! You're the only other man in the house."

"August," I said sarcastically, "if you think I'm manly you *clearly* haven't been paying attention!"

Before anyone could register what I said, Aspen burst into the sunroom. In her hand was a small round Tupperware container.

"I'm gonna catch it and get it outside!" she declared with confidence.

The world went into slow motion as Aspen walked towards the skittish shrew that was still freaking out due to Maggie. Aspen got right on top of her prey and was ready to pounce. The shrew froze and was not sure what to do. She looked at the container, and as fast as she could, Aspen lowered it on top of the shrew.

Unfortunately, the shrew didn't understand that we were going to release it, so it tried to escape. It moved at the last possible second. To our horror, the lip of the container landed right on the shrew's neck, snapping it.

Everyone froze once we processed what just occurred. Aspen looked at the animal that she had just slain, took a deep breath, and yelled at the top of her lungs, "Exterminator!"

CHAPTER 17: THE A-CON SYSTEM
01/21/2011

About a week after the girls and Tina brought me to "Theodora's Woods," Arden texted me while I was at school. It went a little something like this:

Arden: Hey, Mitchie! Do you want to come over tonight and do some videoing for Miracle Child?
Me: Yeah, sure! What time?
Arden: Well, I have to walk Maggie right after school, so maybe around 4:15?
Me: Okay, cool. I will see you then!

I waited until about 4:00 P.M. but then I got tired of waiting. I decided that it was only 15 minutes before Arden would get home, and one of the other girls would be at their house anyway.

When I arrived, Barbara answered the door. "Hey Mitchell," she said as I walked in the house.

"Hey, Barbara," I said. "Is anyone else here?"

"Arden took Maggie on a walk with August and Aspen, but Lo-lo is in the TV room with Shelby."

"Okay, I will just hang with them till the girls get back." I wasn't looking forward to hanging out with Shelby, but I figured if I was going to get this movie made, I shouldn't be mean to her, especially since Arden told me not to be.

I walked into the TV room where Lo-lo and Shelby were playing Jenga. It was obviously very late in the game because the tower was looking precarious.

"Mitchie!" both girls exclaimed.

"Hey guys!" I replied, trying to avoid eye contact with Shelby.

"What are you doing here?" Lo-lo asked.

"The girls and I are going to do some recording for the movie when they get back." Lo-lo and I continued our conversation for about five minutes after this. While we were talking, Shelby thought she could take a few more blocks out of the Jenga tower to make it even more uneven so that when Lo-lo took the next turn, she would lose. She took one too many blocks from the tower, and as a result, it collapsed.

"What the heck, Shelby!" Lo-lo screamed.

"I didn't do anything!" Shelby yelled back, still holding a block in her hand.

"You're lying! You're literally holding the block!" I could see that Lo-lo was fed up with Shelby's crap, and as stated before, I didn't like Shelby either. Even though she was only six years old at the time, I took Lo-lo's side to try to get rid of Shelby.

Lo-lo yelled at Shelby for about 10 minutes before she was ready to kick Shelby out, much to my excitement. It was at this point the other girls returned. Hearing Lo-lo and Shelby arguing, the girls ran into the room. What was said is unnecessary; all that is needed to know is that the older three girls made Lo-lo let Shelby stay.

The night went on after that without incident. I was quite mad that Shelby was still there. When I finally decided to go home, I said goodbye and walked out the side door as I always did. As I departed, Lo-lo ran after me.

"Mitchie!" she whispered as she followed me.

"What?" I asked, confused.

"She's really annoying me. I know she annoys you too. I want to cut her out."

"Yeah, well, we can't really do that, can we? Your sisters definitely won't let us do it."

"Maybe—but I think we could still push her out."

"How?"

"Well, she definitely annoys them. I think the reason they were mad was because I was already hanging out with her. What if we set up a system where if you see her coming, you tell me so I can hide. After a while she's bound to stop coming over."

After a few minutes of talking, I went home and started devising a plan. The plan I came up with was called the "A-con system." If I saw Shelby coming down to the house, I would yell, "A-con 3." The closer she got to the house, the lower the number would get. When Lo-lo would hear the keywords, she would hide, and I would tell Shelby she was not home.

CHAPTER 18: THE LOST SISTER

01/25/2011

One day while the girls and I were setting up to record a scene, Lo-lo saw a picture that she hadn't seen before. Barbara recently had this picture framed. It was of young August sitting next to young Arden, who were holding baby Aspen.

The thing about young Arden is that she looked completely different than she did currently. I don't mean that she grew up and changed a little bit as everyone does. I mean she looked like a completely different person. Because of this fact, of course, when Lo-lo summoned us to the picture and asked who that was, we understood her confusion. What caught us off guard was what August did in response.

"That's our sister… Susie."

"Wait wh--" Arden started only to get cut off.

"She was born between Arden and I," August responded quickly.

"Are you serious!" Lo-lo exclaimed.

"Yeah. See that baby in the picture? That's Arden."

"Where is she now?"

"Well," August began, "one night she got in a big fight with Mom and Dad. She wasn't eating all of her vegetables, and she stormed out of the house mad. After about an hour, we started looking for her. It was like she had just fallen off the face of the earth! We still don't know what happened."

Arden, Aspen, and I looked at each other in shock. We had so many questions and exactly zero answers.

"Why do I not know about this?" Lo-lo asked.

"Mom and Dad just don't talk about it," August said confidently.

Lo-lo thought about it for a second, and after a few moments, she determined that August had to be telling the truth. Arden, Aspen, and I were way too shocked to say anything, giving Lo-lo even more reason to believe that she had a fourth sister.

CHAPTER 19: THE MAKEOVER

02/01/2011

"How are we going to open the movie?" The girls asked me a few days later.

"What do you mean?"

"Well," Arden said, "I had to do a movie project about a year ago, and I did a clip at the beginning explaining what the movie was about. I think that would be a nice touch."

Within the next 10 minutes, I was sitting in the sunroom with Arden's video camera in my face, and all four girls crowded around me. "What do you want me to say?" I asked.

"Just introduce yourself and tell people about the movie!" Arden said.

"Okay um--" I said.

"You can start." Arden hit the record button, and I took a deep breath. "Hey everybody, it's John Mitchell Ulibarri! What you're about to watch is the movie I made with my friends for the 'HLC Make a Movie Project.' I hope you enjoy and have an awesome day!"

"That was good--" Aspen started.

"But?" Lo-lo asked.

"It's just missing a little flair!"

August and Arden looked at each other with intense excitement. Suddenly August and Arden pulled me out of the chair, led me upstairs, chanting, "Makeover, Makeover, Makeover!" Lo-lo joined the chant, and followed us upstairs, while I wondered what I'd gotten myself into. We walked into Aspen and Lo-lo's room. The girls started talking amongst themselves and Arden entered the room with a speaker and her mom's iPhone.

"We can't have a makeover without music!" she exclaimed as the music started playing.

Arden's playlist consisted of artists such as Justin Bieber, Miley Cyrus (more accurately Hannah Montana), One Direction, and the Jonas Brothers, and Taylor Swift. In fact, Taylor Swift's entire album "Fearless" was on the playlist. As the girls were giving me this makeover, I would take any chance I got to make fun of the artists.

"All of Taylor Swift's music is the same!" I would say in annoyance.

"No, it's not!" the girls retorted.

"Guys," I said insolently, "they're all about a guy she's in love with, or a guy who broke her heart!"

"Wow," said August. "Someone's sassy."

I winked at her and said, "Duh!" I probably shouldn't have said that because the girls got a little more aggressive with the makeover after that. It happened so fast that I didn't know what was going on. All I knew was that suddenly I was wearing a pink dress and a blond wig.

Eventually Barbara came up the stairs confused. "What did you do to this boy?"

"Nothing--" August said as the other girls looked away.

"Mitchell, get that off!"

I got the dress off, and we all walked downstairs. When Rich got home from work, he instituted a rule: no boys upstairs ever!

CHAPTER 20: THE JONES FRACTURE

02/07/2011

About a year before I went to school at Haugland, a few of the Duck Clan members wanted to play basketball for OLP. The members who wanted to join asked the rest of the group if they also wanted to join. The problem was that Ryan tended to overthink often. He had never played basketball, which made him overthink this decision. Ultimately, decisions like this stressed him out.

Knowing that Ryan was struggling with this decision, my parents decided to give him a pep talk one night at dinner. I don't remember what was said, exactly, but by the end of the night, Ryan felt a little better about the decision and soon after decided to join the team.

Somehow or another, Dad got dragged into becoming a coach for the team. He started to watch basketball games, and he studied the positions. After he memorized all the game positions, he grew to be a fantastic coach and led the team to many victories.

On Super Bowl Sunday, Ryan's basketball team had a late-night practice in the school gym. Dad unlocked the door to the gym, and the kids started to pour into the gym, followed immediately by the second coach.

"Line up boys!" the other coach said. The boys fell into position, and he continued. "Tonight, we're going to have a scrimmage. I'll be on one team and Mr. Ulibarri will be on the other!" They put the teams together, and Ryan and Dad ended up on the same team.

The first few plays went by without incident, but tragedy struck around the fourth or fifth play. Ryan got the ball but was surrounded by the other team. He looked around and saw that Dad was open, so he passed the ball to him.

Dad dribbled the ball around a few kids and got to the three-point line only to be surrounded by kids reaching for the ball. Dad jumped in the air, shot the ball, and made the basket. Dad came down from the jump and immediately felt an unbearable pain in his foot. He hobbled to the sidelines and sat out for the rest of the practice.

The next morning, Mom took me to school then immediately took Dad to the doctor. He had what is called a Jones Fracture. The doctor told him that it would take about 11 weeks to heal. During that time, he would have to be in a boot and walk on crutches.

Of course, this produced a few problems: For starters, Dad rides his bike to work every day, and because of his foot, he couldn't do that. As a result, he was frustrated. The more significant issue was that it would be a lot harder for him to manage all of his employees because he would not be able to run around his studio checking up on them all the time.

Dad had been keeping his family updated on what was happening at the doctor's office. After hearing the diagnosis and the healing time, Pop-Pop decided to come to Ohio and help Dad out with the studio until he was back on his feet (pun intended).

Pop-Pop had a few jobs that he had to finish over the next three weeks, so he couldn't fly up until he had finished. Those three weeks would end up changing the course of my relationship with the Andersons!

CHAPTER 21: THE WAY IT WILL BE

02/08/2011

As a result of Dad's broken foot and the doctor's appointment, Dad was late getting to the studio. Work had backed up throughout the time that Dad was gone, meaning that he and Mom had to play catch-up. OLP was only about a mile from our house, so the boys were able to walk home. I could not walk home because Haugland was much farther away. Mom texted Barbara and asked her if she could pick me up.

Arden had Tina over when Mom texted Barbara, who was about to run errands anyway. Upon hearing that I needed to get picked up, Arden and Tina decided to come along. They picked me up in the family's gold minivan, nicknamed by the girls "Old Betsy."

"Hey Mitchie!" both girls exclaimed from the back seat when I entered.

"Hey!" I replied, excited to see them both.

"So, we are going to OfficeMax before we head home. Is that okay?" Barbara asked me.

"Yeah, that's fine!"

When we pulled up to the store, I looked back at the girls and saw that Tina was smiling. As we exited "Old Betsy," Tina put her arm around my shoulder and whispered in my ear, "Follow my lead."

We walked into the store, and Barbara started shopping. We arrived at an aisle when Tina asked a question that would change the day. "Hey, Mrs.

Anderson," she asked, "can Arden, Mitchie, and I go walk around the store?"

"Sure, where are you going to go?"

"We're not really sure, we just wanna look around. We will stay in the store." Arden explained.

"Okay," Barbara replied. "Meet me at the front of the store in 15 minutes."

"Awesome, thanks!" both girls exclaimed as they started to run off. "Come on Mitchie!"

"Coming!"

"And don't do anything stupid," Barbara called after us, anticipating the shenanigans that were about to come.

We walked around the store, goofed off, and just had a good time. Eventually, we turned a corner and saw a small carpeted area. A few shelves were lining the walls in the area. In the middle of the carpet were three rolling chairs just waiting for our arrival.

"Are you guys thinking what I'm thinking?" Tina asked.

"Absolutely!" Arden replied with a grin.

We lined up the chairs, one in front of the other. Arden sat in the front chair, Tina in the back, and I took the middle. I put my hands on the back of Arden's chair, and Tina did the same to mine. We then propelled our makeshift train with our feet.

The problem was, of course, that there were three of us. That's three different pairs of feet trying to propel three separate rolling chairs in one direction. Every time we tried to make a turn, we would crash into a wall or shelf.

"Hey!" I said after a great deal of destruction was made. "We obviously can't control ourselves together, so why don't we try rolling around on our own?"

The girls agreed, and we changed our tactic. We all knelt on our seats and pushed ourselves like you would on a scooter. We sped through the whole store, crashing into each other and laughing the entire time. Tina got a little bit ahead of Arden, who then tried to get in front of Tina. The two viciously tried to pass one another, unintentionally starting a race. I didn't want to get left behind, so I sped up and tried to keep up with them.

The longer this race went on meant the farther I got left behind. The adrenaline started pumping through me, and I didn't care about anything except catching up with the girls. Unfortunately, this way of thinking clouded my judgment, and so I pushed a little too hard, flipped over the back of the chair, and flew through the air. When I crashed to the floor, all of the air left my body. The girls, hearing the crash, turned around to see what had happened.

"Oh my gosh! Mitchie, are you okay?" Arden asked in a panicked voice.

"Never… been… better!" I said between gasps.

"Oh my gosh," Arden said, rolling her eyes. "Come on, let's go before you hurt yourself even more."

"Yeah…that would probably be a good idea!" Tina agreed.

We found Barbara when she was about to check out. "Ah, there you are!" she said when she saw us. "I was just about to text you!"

The girls and I looked at each other. Smiles slowly crept across our faces, and simultaneously we burst into laughter. We did not stop laughing until we got to "Old Betsy."

"Okay, what's so funny?" Barbara asked as we started to drive away. We explained what had happened. As the story progressed, we just laughed harder and harder. As we drove home, I imagined what my life would be like with the girls in the future.

***

"Daddy, Daddy!" my daughter yelled, jumping onto my and Caroline's bed. "It's time to get up, everyone's coming over today!"

"Sam," I yawned as I looked over at the clock, "it's literally 6:30."

"They're coming over at 8:00! And I still need to eat breakfast!"

"You see them every day. Can't we be late just this once?"

"No, Daddy," Sam said, giggling. "You say that every morning!"

"Like father, like daughter," Caroline groaned.

"Y... y... you... shut up!"

Caroline rolled over, "Well good morning to you too!"

I got up, got dressed, made Sam breakfast, got her dressed, and waited for everyone to arrive. When they all came, the kids started playing together while we adults began talking about the things that were going on in our lives. After about an hour playing, Sam and the other kids walked up to us.

"Daddy," Sam asked me, "how did you guys meet and become close friends?" I looked at the girls, and they looked back at me.

I smiled and said, "It all started with a movie--"

***

When we got home, the biggest smile stretched across my face. I knew this relationship that I had been building with these girls went far beyond this stupid "school project." I truly believed that we would be hanging out for the rest of our lives to the point where all of our kids would be best friends.

CHAPTER 22: THE BOX OF LOVE NOTES
02/12/2011-02/14/2011

As soon as Caroline and Jake started dating, I started avoiding them. The good news was my time with their group, and the "Dr. Mitch" stuff had made me popular enough that the whole school was my friend group. The bad news was my feelings for Caroline didn't go away just because I was avoiding her; in fact, this avoidance made them stronger. As if things couldn't get any worse, Valentine's Day was fast approaching.

On February 12th, while we were recording *Miracle Child*, I was very distracted because I knew Valentine's Day was two days away. I was not looking forward to going to school.

"Mitchie," Arden asked, stopping the recording. "What's wrong?"

"Yeah, you're acting really strange," Aspen added.

"It's nothing," I said in a dry tone.

"Come on, tell us!" August exclaimed.

"So basically, there's this girl at school, but she has a boyfriend and I'm just not looking forward to Valentine's Day because of that."

The girls tried to comfort me, but it was pretty clear that everything they were doing was not helping the situation. Eventually, I told them that I would be fine and that we should continue recording.

***

After school on the following day, when I walked into the Andersons' kitchen, I saw all four Anderson girls, plus Melody and Shelby, sitting at the kitchen table with a bunch of construction paper scraps in front of them. In their hands were either some coloring utensils or zig-zag scissors.

"Noooooooo!" They all yelled when they saw me. Everyone told me that I had to leave, and that I could come back the next day.

Confused, I walked out of the house. Without the girls, I knew I wouldn't be able to distract myself from the whole Caroline predicament. As I walked back towards my house, Greg stepped out of his front door.

"Hey Mitchell!" he called, running up to me.

"Greg!" I exclaimed, excited to see him. We had not seen each other in close to a month and a half, so we started catching up. Of course, I brought up Caroline and how I was feeling about that.

"Aw, dude," he uttered sympathetically. "That really stinks! Personally, I'm also going through something like that at the moment." As soon as those words left his mouth, a look of regret fell across his face.

"What's wrong?" I asked.

"Well it's just--," he started, "you have to promise you won't tell the girls what I'm about to tell you."

"Okay?" I said, baffled.

"I have a crush on August, but I know she doesn't like me back, so I don't want to say anything." I was genuinely shocked by this realization. I promised that I wouldn't tell the girls this secret.

***

Valentine's Day 2011 was as I expected it to be, a total downer. Nothing went my way at school, and all I wanted to do was go home. Luckily for me, when I did get home, my day picked up.

As Mom was pulling into the driveway, I noticed pink balloons on my front porch. I asked her if she knew anything about them, and she told me she didn't. When I proceeded inside through the back door, I ran through the house and opened the front door.

The balloon ribbon was tied around a reddish-pink box covered in stars. There were two white paper strips taped on top of the box, followed by a thick piece of red duct tape and a final white paper strip. From top to bottom, the strips read as follows:

Paper strip 1: Mitchell ONLY
Paper strip 2: Special Delivery
Red duct tape: Mitchell
Paper strip 3: FRAGILE

I took the box along with the balloon inside and opened it. The box's inside was filled with the scraps of construction paper cut out with zig-zag scissors and a ton of Hershey's Kisses. On the inside lid, there was a message that read:

Dear Mitchell:
HAPPY VALENTINES DAY!!
Here are a few things that make you great...
...make sure to read ALL of them!

I poured the contents out of the box, onto the kitchen table, and read the scraps of construction paper:

VERY ENTERTAINING.
You are special.
Thanks for caring about me!
Dear Mitchell: I+God=love you sooo much.
Mitchell: Sorry for when we were mean to you!
You are so sweet; you knock me off my feet!
You're one in a million.
You make me laugh.
Mitchie, you make my day.
You bring joy to others!!
You have a big heart!
You are so awesome!
You only think of the good in people.
You are amazing, special, considerate, smart, cool, awesome- words can't describe you!

There are about 50 more, but I think I have made my point. I ran as fast as I could over to the Andersons' house. When I entered, the Anderson girls, Shelby and Melody, greeted me with a loud, "Happy Valentine's Day!"

"Guys?" I asked. "Why did you do that?"

"Because it's what friends do! We pick each other up when they're feeling down!" Arden replied.

"Friends," I repeated aloud, confirming that I had made friends and that the hard part was over. Unfortunately, the hard part was only beginning.

CHAPTER 23: THE END OF BLISS

06/19/1978-02/24/2011

In the late 70s, a girl by the name of Renee was born in Tokyo, Japan. From a very young age, Renee was a very driven person. When she was 19 years old, she found a stray black and white cat named him Marble and claimed him as her own. Soon after that, she taught herself English by using a Japanese to English dictionary and moved to Columbus to go to school at The Ohio State University. Her dream was to become a piano teacher. Over time she earned her doctorate. She met a man named Rob in school, and the two ended up getting married.

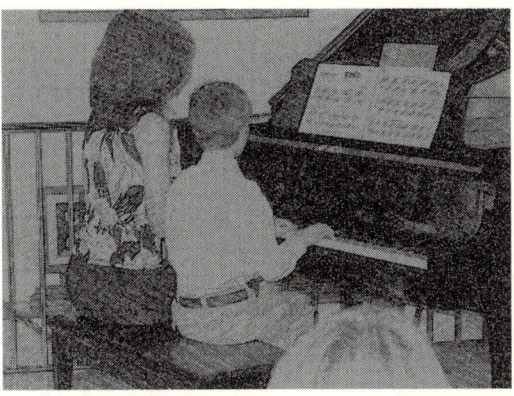

Back during our fairytale childhood, August, Arden, Ryan, and I took piano lessons from a woman, who... how do I say this? Well, she was very strict, to say the least. Not that that's necessarily a bad thing. The problem was that when I was a kid, I didn't have the discipline needed to learn how to play an instrument. I dreaded practice every week because I didn't do all my homework. Even in the weeks I practiced tirelessly, it wasn't good enough, and she would still yell, "Shame on you!" while slapping me on the head with my *Music Theory* book. As a result, all of us eventually stopped learning the piano.

Shortly after the fairytale ended, August started piano lessons again under the tutelage of Renee. On top of this, the lessons were completely free because Barbara and the girls watched Renee's one-and-a-half-year-old daughter, Hotaru, when Renee taught students on Wednesdays and Thursdays.

I walked over to the Andersons' house on Thursday, two weeks after Dad broke his foot. I walked into the kitchen and heard August on the piano. Barbara dashed into the kitchen, shushing me with her finger.

"August is in the middle of her piano lesson," she explained in a whisper. "The others are outside playing on the trampoline."

I made a goofy smile, gave her a thumbs-up, and ran out to the backyard. Arden, Aspen, Lo-lo, and Shelby were sitting on the trampoline with Hotaru. Maggie was waiting right outside the trampoline for everyone to get out so she could play. She spotted me approaching the trampoline, and out of excitement, ran up to me and started barking.

"Hey, guys!" I said while petting Maggie.

"Mitchie!" the girls yelled.

Hotaru was taken aback by the loud noise and my sudden appearance. Aspen knelt and explained to her that I was not a threat. For about 10 minutes after that, we played outside and tried to distract Hotaru from going inside. Hotaru was talkative and very energetic, which made distracting her almost effortless. The girls seemed very protective of her, a sentiment I would eventually adopt.

"Awden," Hotaru said, "I want snack! "

"Can you be quiet while we are inside?" Arden asked the toddler.

"Yes!"

We moved into the house and got Hotaru settled. As she had her snack, we listened to August play. She finished a song, and Renee told her how good of a job she did.

"How are you doing on 'You're not Sorry'?" Renee asked.

"I'll show you!" August replied. There was a pause, and then she started playing the song.

I had heard the song a few times before but only in Taylor Swift's voice, not August's. When August sang it, it felt directed at me as opposed to an ex-lover.

I started to panic because, at that moment, I realized that I didn't ever want the girls to get so mad at me and risk ending our friendship. I could see our future slowly fading away—the future where we all grow up together and see our kids become best friends. I knew I had to do anything and everything in my power to keep that almost inevitable fate from occurring.

CHAPTER 24: THE KISS
02/24/2011-02/28/2011

I didn't get much sleep that night because I could not keep my frightening thoughts at bay. I needed to stop thinking about what the girls might do if they ever found out I was lying to them about the movie. I knew that they probably wouldn't be able to forgive me for it. Our relationship would undeniably go back to the way it was before we started making the movie. I thought telling them the truth at this point wouldn't help either because regardless of how our friendship was, they would feel betrayed.

I had crafted a plan by the end of the night: finish the movie, let our families watch it, and then let it collect dust on a shelf. The girls would eventually forget about it, and we could move on with our lives. There was still a problem, even though I came up with what seemed to be a flawless solution, the guilt continued to eat me up.

When I went to the Andersons' house to record the next day, we only had a few more scenes left before we finished the movie. Every time Arden turned that video camera on, I froze up because I knew that I was hurting them without them knowing.

"What's wrong with you today?" Aspen asked.

"Nothing," I snapped back at her.

"We know there's something wrong," August said. "You're not acting like yourself." The girls looked at each other and then at me.

"Mitchie," Arden started hesitantly, "have you been lying to us?"

"No, I haven't!" I said a little too loudly.

"Oh my gosh, yes you have been!" Lo-lo yelled.

The girls were piecing everything together. I knew I had only seconds to save everything. I took a deep breath, and with confidence, said, "No I haven't, and I can prove it."

"How?" the girls asked collectively.

"My teacher gave all of the kids in the class an instruction sheet. I can show it to you."

"Why is this the first we've heard about this sheet?" August asked.

"It wasn't important until now."

"Fine!" Aspen scoffed. "Go get it!"

I sprinted home as fast as I could. I opened the back door and ran to the basement. "Yes!" I exclaimed when I saw no one was on the computer. I typed up fake instructions for how we should make this movie.

I was about to print it off when I remembered one crucial detail. When Derek would send something home, he would sign his name at the bottom of whatever he was sending. I knew at this point, the girls didn't know that, but I was thinking ahead. If Derek sent something home signed and the girls saw it in the future, it would nullify the fake document I had just written up.

I told the girls that I had forgotten the document on my desk at school, but I would bring it to them when I went back to school on Monday. I would explain the situation to Derek, he would understand and sign the document, and everything would be okay.

***

I got to school early on Monday in an attempt to get Derek alone. Max somehow managed to get there before me, so I decided to explain everything to Derek at lunch.

I walked into the lunchroom, set all my stuff down on the table by Max, and told him I would be right back. As I was walking to Derek's room with the instructions in hand, Caroline saw me and started following me at a distance.

When I got to the room, Derek was not there. I was under pressure, so I decided to sign it myself as Derek. I sat down at his desk, grabbed a pencil, and just when I was about to sign, Caroline walked in the door.

"Hey Mitch, what are you doing?"

"Nothing." I said, slightly annoyed that she was there.

"Come on Mitch," she coaxed, "we're still friends, right?"

"Yeah of course." I said shortly.

"Then come on, tell me!" At that, I buckled and told her everything. "Wow!" she exclaimed when I had finished, "You've gotten yourself into quite a pickle. Here let me help."

"What are you doing?" I asked as she took the pencil out of my hand.

"I'm signing that for you. They might recognize your handwriting."

"True," I agreed.

"So," she asked as she signed Derek's name, "why have you been avoiding me?"

"What? I haven't been avoiding you!" I lied.

"Come on Mitch!" she said, rolling her eyes. "Ever since Jake and I became a couple, you haven't been sitting with us or talking to us. You don't even text me anymore! What happened?"

"I mean, nothing happened--" I said, avoiding eye contact, "You know just sometimes… friendships don't work out I guess--"

"Do you want our friendship to end?"

"No! But…" I trailed off.

"Mitch," she said, looking into my eyes, "I know. I know everything. It's so obvious."

"What's obvious?" I asked.

She didn't answer the question. She stayed silent, but in that silence was something I had never heard before. Even though she wasn't saying anything, I could almost hear what she was thinking. I wanted to do it too, so I kissed her.

Unfortunately, there was a problem. No, not the fact that Caroline had a boyfriend, though we will get to that. No, the problem was that I still felt guilty about what had happened with the last girl I liked.

CHAPTER 25: THE GIRL OF MY DREAMS
08/26/2003-02/28/2011

On the first day of kindergarten, I was feeling homesick. At recess, on that day, it all came to a head, and I became depressed. One of my classmates noticed that I was having a rough time. "Are you okay?" she asked.

"Yes," I said, embarrassed.

"I'm Samantha," she said, "but you can call me Sam."

"I'm Mitchell," I replied.

"Do you want to talk?"

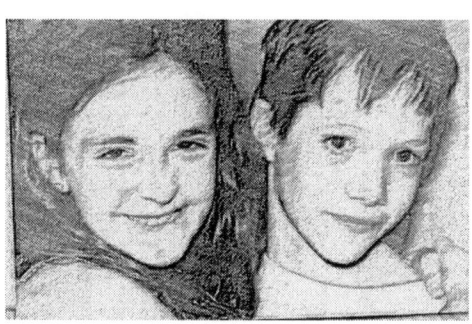

That's how our friendship began. I eventually gave Sam the nickname S.M. because those are her initials. As the years went on, I developed a major crush on S.M. Because I was so young and still incredibly self-conscious, I did not tell her anything.

Unfortunately for me, in third grade, S.M.'s family decided to move across town. As a result, she had to change schools. I was distraught on the last day of school that year. As I was walking to Mom's car, I saw a group of girls from my class standing around S.M, and they were all crying. S.M. looked up, saw me, walked out of the middle of the group, and motioned for me to meet her.

"Hi," I said when I got to her.

"I'm going to miss you!" S.M. said, hugging me.

"I'd miss me too!" I said, trying to be funny, but only managing to make myself feel sadder.

"It's going to be okay, we'll still see each other" S.M. said with a smile.

We didn't see each other until the end of the summer. My birthday party that year was at a swimming pool, and I invited S.M. We picked up exactly where we left off, and it was magical! After the party, she came to my house for a little bit before her mom arrived to pick her up. Shortly before her mom got to my house, we decided to grab a snack.

"Do you want a granola bar?" I asked when we got to the cabinet.

"Sure!"

"Good, cuz that's the only thing we have!" I said, throwing the bar at her.

"Ouch!" she exclaimed when it hit her in the face.

"Oh my gosh! I'm so sorry!"

"Mitchell, it's fine!" she said, laughing. I still felt awful about it. When I kept freaking out about it, she looked at me and said, "You're so cute... I could kiss you right now!"

***

You're so cute I could kiss you right now! The words echoed in my head as I pushed Caroline away. "Sorry," I said to her.

"What's wrong?"

"That was." I said.

"Why?"

"Well, you have a boyfriend, and I kind of have a girlfriend."

"What do you mean 'kind of' have a girlfriend?!" Caroline asked angrily.

"There was this girl… I was in love with her, but now she's gone."

"She's gone?"

I took a long pause because I wasn't sure how much I should tell her. I eventually decided *not* to tell her everything. "She moved away," I said dryly.

"So, you're still a couple, even though she moved?"

"I mean, no, but--"

"Then what's the problem?"

"Look, it's just really complicated, okay? We never really ended things and on top of that, you have a boyfriend, who is one of my friends!"

It was at this point that the weight of the situation hit her. "What do we do?" she asked.

I thought for a second. I knew what we did was wrong, but I also knew that it wasn't as the worst thing in the world. It was just a kiss, one time, for five seconds. "Let's just pretend this never happened," I offered. "It was just a kiss; he doesn't have to know about it. No one needs to get hurt."

While I was still talking, Jake walked into the room, and he glared at both of us. "What are you guys doing?!"

"Jake--" Caroline started.

"Shut up!" he replied, as he charged at me. He put his hands on my chest and pushed me up against the wall.

"Jake, stop it!" Caroline pleaded.

"Mitch," he said, "I don't ever want to see you guys together again, and our friendship is over!"

With that, he pulled Caroline out of the room. As soon as they left, I grabbed the document and stormed out of the room.

I was distraught. I was mad at Jake for disowning me. I was mad that Caroline and I had kissed, and that it went so badly. But I was mostly mad because I put myself in this situation. I lied to the girls; I'd snuck into a teacher's room to keep the lie going. And as a result, I was now losing friends at school. If S.M was with me right then, I knew she would have been disappointed.

But I knew I couldn't stop, especially after these events. I had lost my main friend group at school, so the girls were all I had left.

SEASON 3: THE MIRACLE WAR

CHAPTER 26: THE GIRL IN THE WINDOW
02/28/2011-03/07/2011

On the ride back from school that day, I was quiet. When we were about halfway home, Mom asked me what was wrong. I told her nothing was wrong, but I needed to get home as soon as possible. I knew the sooner I got home, the sooner I could give the document to the girls, and then we could finish the movie, and then put this whole situation behind us.

"Wow!" August said when I showed the document to the girls, "We honestly thought you were lying for a hot second there!"

"Who, me?" I said, trying not to look as nervous as I was, "Why would I lie to you guys?"

Everyone laughed, and we got back to work finishing the movie. By Friday of that week, we had finished recording and put the finished product onto a DVD. On the top of the disc, the girls wrote words of encouragement and love for me using multi-colored markers.

"You know what we should do!" Arden exclaimed when they had finished writing on the DVD.

"What?" We all asked in unison.

"Tomorrow we should all go over to the Ulibarri's house, and show it to your family, before you give it to your teacher!"

"Oh my gosh, that's a really good idea!" Aspen exclaimed, and the other girls agreed.

Now, I had told my family that I was working on a movie with the girls, but I had not told them about how I had convinced the girls to make it. I did not think it would be too big of a deal, though. I would never let my family be alone with the girls, and I was confident in my ability to steer the conversation away from the movie being a school project. Unfortunately, I had forgotten about one particular clip.

At 10:00 the next morning, the girls came over to my house, with the disc in hand. After a little bit of small talk, we popped the movie in, and we sat on the couch.

I appeared on the TV, sitting in the Andersons' sunroom. "Hey everybody, it's John Mitchell Ulibarri!" TV Mitchell announced. "What you're about to watch is the movie I made with my friends for the 'HLC Make a Movie project.' I hope you enjoy and have an awesome day!"

My heart started pounding. I didn't know what to do. If anyone said anything, my tangled web of lies would be exposed! Both of my parents looked at me, and I slowly brought my finger to my lips. They both still had confused expressions on their faces. To my surprise, the girls didn't start questioning me or even glare at me. As we watched, I *assumed* that they hadn't noticed.

When the movie was over, my family cheered and told us that it was "Awesome!"

"Thank you." Arden said, standing up, "Mitchie, will you be over later today?"

"No, Pop-pop is coming in about an hour, and I'm going to spend time with him today."

"Okay, see you later. Come on, girls," Arden replied.

When they were out the door, I let out a sigh of relief, not knowing the trouble that was about to start.

***

The following Monday, when I got home, I went straight to the kitchen and grabbed a quick after-school snack. I was planning to go hang out with the girls after my snack. As I ate, Will, Ryan, Luke, Josh came up from the basement.

"Hey guys." I said when I saw them.

"Hey Mitchell." They all replied.

"How was school?"

"It was good," Ryan said. "I told Will about your movie."

"Really?"

"Yeah," Will replied, "Could I see it?"

"Sure, why not!"

We went to the TV room and started the movie. The TV room had five windows on the wall. Three of them were directly across from the TV. Out of those three, the only thing visible was the fence that divided our yard and the Andersons' yard. The other two faced the circle, which could be seen, but there was a big bushy tree in front of it. The couch was directly under the three windows facing the fence and next to the circle's window. Will and my three brothers sat down, I popped in the DVD, and we started watching. About halfway through the movie, I got a text from Arden. Here's our conversation:

Arden: Hey Mitchie, R U coming over today?
Me: Yeah. I'll be over soon!
Arden: How soon?
Me: Idk... 20 mins
Arden: What R you doing right now?
Me: Not Much
Arden: Really?

No sooner had I read the question "Really?" when there was an angry banging at the window facing the circle. We all jumped, and Luke let out a scream. Out the window right under the tree, glaring at me, was Lo-lo!

CHAPTER 27: THE DISK

03/07/2011

We all sat there, shocked at the little girl staring at us. Lo-lo continued to bang on the window. "Come outside right now, Mitchell!" she ordered. I walked out my front door and saw August, Arden, Aspen, and Shelby, waiting at my front porch.

"So, you did lie to us!" August yelled as Lo-lo came around the corner of my house.

"Guys--" I said, trying to explain myself.

"No, you don't get to talk!" Aspen interrupted. "Why were you showing it to them?"

"I didn't think it would be a problem. It's not like I posted it anywhere!"

"Well it is a problem!" August scoffed.

"I just don't understand why you lied to all of us!" Shelby said.

"You know what, shut up Shelby!" I snapped. "This doesn't concern you!"

"Well, she's right!" Lo-lo defended. "Why were you lying to us?"

"You know what Arlo; don't you dare defend her! You are the one who came to me and told me that you didn't like her okay!"

Everyone looked at Lo-lo, completely shocked, while she just glared at me. Shelby ran off crying, and Lo-lo ran to comfort her.

"Wow, real mature Mitchell!" Arden said, turning and leading the other two girls away.

"I didn't do anything wrong!" I yelled.

117

"You didn't do anything wrong?" August turned around, "You lied to us, wasted our time, you just made Shelby cry, and worst of all you won't tell us why you lied?"

"You want to know why I lied? Really? I lied because of you! I was lonely, I wanted to spend time with anybody, and we used to be good friends, so I thought you were my best shot! I knew you guys would not do it if I didn't lie to you! If anything, this is your fault because you guys started this mess when you shot Will in the eye with soap water!"

"That was years ago Mitchell!" Arden cried, her back still turned to me, "We didn't mean for this to get so out of hand, but you're the one who's making it worse! You're the one who always makes it worse!"

The girls walked inside and left me outside to fume. I was so mad they were angry at me when they were the ones who not only started everything but then would pretend like I didn't exist whenever they thought I did something wrong.

I stormed to the shed and unlocked the door. I searched around for a second and found Ryan's water gun. I ran into the house, put soap in the gun, and then filled it up with water.

"What are you doing?" Ryan asked

"They started it like this," I said slyly, "and that's how I'm going to finish it!"

I ran to the Andersons' house, and I stood outside and just started squirting the outside of the house. I hit windows, some siding, nothing significant considering that it was just soap and water; I cleaned the house more or less. The problem was this was early March, so it was still kind of cold. Barbara came out, and she was furious.

"What are you doing!?" she yelled.

"Nothing." I said coolly.

"You're going to wipe all this off the house right now!"

I rolled my eyes, which in hindsight, was not the best response. Barbara raised an eyebrow at me, and I knew I should do what she said, or I was going to get into trouble. Barbara led me into the house and handed me a roll of paper towels. As I was walking back out the door, all of the girls were glaring at me.

After I had dried off the house, I went back inside to put the paper towels back. The three oldest girls stood behind their mother, still giving me the evil eye. I could hear Lo-lo and Shelby shouting upstairs. Barbara looked at me, and a stern look fell across her face.

"Mitchell," she said, "you're going to walk over to your house, grab the movie, and give it back to the girls."

"Why should I?"

"Because you lied to them, and you hurt them."

"I only lied because--"

"I don't want to hear it." Barbara interrupted. "Why you did it doesn't matter. What matters is they are hurt!"

I realized that they were not going to listen to anything I was going to say, so I decided to concede defeat. I unhappily marched over to my house, escorted by August and Aspen.

"Here you go," I grumbled as I handed the disk over to August.

"Thanks," August replied sarcastically.

Without another word, the two walked back to their house, with the disc in hand. A wave of sadness washed over me. I walked into my room, as calmly as I could, sat down on my bed, and started crying.

CHAPTER 28: THE MIRACLE WAR BEGINS
03/11/2011

The next Friday, my family had a few people over to see Pop-pop. The guest list consisted of the Crawfords, Anita and Ron Wallace, and their two children Tanner and Maya. Everyone was so excited to see Pop-pop because they didn't get to see him too much.

At dinner, as usual, Pop-pop started telling stories. Most of them were awkward situations that he had just recently gotten himself into, but one involved Dad. In response to the Dad story, Anita and Ron started telling a couple of stories from when my parents were back in college with them.

As a writer (or when I was younger, just a storyteller), I have an uncontrollable need to name stories. It just feels more real if a story has a name associated with it. Anyways, the stories that Anita and Ron were telling us were called "The Adventures of Danger Boy and Panic Girl."

Most of the stories were structured with Dad deciding to do something crazy. Mom's immediate response was always along the lines of, "Jerry get down from there!" or, "Jerry be careful!" Anita and Ron would then laugh at the situation. Everyone at the table was cracking up because the nicknames "Danger Boy and Panic Girl" are the perfect names to describe my parents, even to this day.

Even though I was laughing at this, these stories made me sad. All I wanted was to have friends--that was it. I wanted to have kids and tell the same kind of stories about my friends to my kids. But not only were things falling apart at school, but now the girls were mad at me, and I just felt so alone.

I went outside after dinner because we are getting closer to springtime, and it was beautiful out. I sat in the circle, enjoying the fresh air. Megan followed me outside, and we started talking. As our conversation went on, I explained what had happened with the girls. I also expressed that I had been bored that week because I didn't have anyone to hang out with after school.

"You have Netflix, right?" Megan asked.

"Yeah," I said. "Any good shows that you know of?"

"I can think of a few."

"Do you want to watch something?" I asked

"Sure!"

Now at this point, we had been talking for about 10 minutes. During that time, August and Aspen had come outside. As Megan and I walked back towards my house, they called out to her.

"Why are you hanging out with *him?!*" they called.

"What did you just say!?" I yelled, starting to feel my face get hot.

"You heard us!" August replied. "Why would anyone want to hang out with you?"

"I'm warning you, Megan," Aspen continued, "he's just going to stab you in the back! That's what he did to us!"

"Oh, shut up!" I exclaimed, "I only had to lie to you guys because--"

"We told you before it doesn't matter!" August yelled. "We let you into our Sisterhood... into our family... and you lied to us!"

There were so many things I wanted to say, but I knew if I tried to say any of them, I would cry, and I didn't want to look weak, so I lied. "Well you know what," I screamed, holding back the tears. "I didn't want to be in your stupid 'Sisterhood' anyway!" I then calmly walked back to my house, walked up to my room, closed the door behind me, and started crying.

As the tears streamed down my face, I looked under my bed and saw the reddish-pink box that the girls had given me for Valentine's Day. I opened the box and started looking over the kind words that the girls had said about me, trying to confirm for myself that somewhere deep down, they still felt the same way. Suddenly the door opened, and Greg walked into my room.

"What are you doing here?" I asked him, wiping the tears away from my face.

"I was eating dinner, and my front window was opened, and I heard you yelling, and I just wanted to check on you. You okay?" I explained what had happened over the past week and how upset the girls were making me.

"I mean they kicked me out of the group and took the disc. I don't have their friendship anymore and I have nothing to show for my effort. I deserve something!"

Greg sat there a moment, pondering what he could do to help me. After a few minutes, he hugged me and then started to talk.

"Yeah that really sucks I'm so sorry Mitchell. But you can't let them win! If you're crying about it, and you are feeling bad about it, then it's just taking more away from you, not fixing the problem. If you want the problem fixed, fix it! What do you want to do? I will help you with whatever it is."

I thought about it for a second. I wanted to be that friend, but I wasn't going to admit that. I thought it was an insane wish. Why would they even consider being my friend again? I barely convinced them the first time! I thought if I couldn't have them, I would get that disc, and I knew exactly how we were going to do it.

"Let's get that disk!" I declared.

"How?"

"Let's just annoy them, until they give it to us!"

"What?"

"Think about it," I said, smiling. "If we annoy them enough, and pick enough fights with them, they'll eventually get tired of the fighting. To make it stop they will give us anything we want!"

Greg thought about this for a second. He seemed a little hesitant. At the time, I believed it was because of his feelings for August, which was partially correct. Still, I think the morality of the situation was an even more significant part of it. Despite all of that, he knew I was hurting, and he didn't know how else to help me, so he decided to play along.

CHAPTER 29: THE RUNAWAY DOG
3/14/2011

The first thing I did when I got home from school that next Monday was text Greg:

Are You home from school?
Yep!
Awesome! Meet me in my backyard ASAP!

"Are you sure you want to do this?" Greg asked when he saw me waiting.

"Yes!" I said, obviously frustrated.

"Okay okay!" He replied defensively, "How are we going to do this?"

"You walk through the driveway and enter the backyard by the garage and then hide. I will hop the fence and start jumping on the trampoline. The girls will see me and come to kick me out. As they are leading me out, you come out of your hiding place and you start jumping on the trampoline. Then we keep it going as long as we can."

"Okay! Let's do this!" he said, walking towards the front yard.

"Text me when you're in position!" I called.

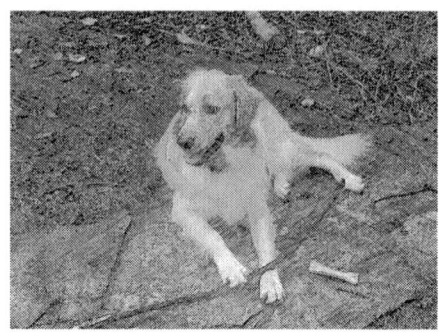

I was very excited and incredibly proud of myself for coming up with such a plan. I knew that it wouldn't get me the disk right away, but I thought it was a good start. There was, unfortunately, something I hadn't been thinking about when I devised the plan: Maggie.

Greg told me he was in position, and I got to work. Now, the side of the fence that faced my yard was the backside of the fence, with the horizontal beams running across it, while the side in the Andersons' yard was the smooth front side.

I hopped the fence and stood on the Andersons' side, my heart pounding. The trampoline was about a hundred feet away from me. All I had to do was make it to the trampoline without any detection, so the girls couldn't stop the plan before we could start it. I surveyed the yard one last time before I made my move and took a double take. Maggie was standing on the back porch, staring right at me.

Maggie wasn't a vicious dog; she was a very kind and loving animal. I think when she saw me, she recognized me and wanted to play. Before I could register what was happening, Maggie started barking and running towards me. I grabbed the top of the fence and tried to pull myself up, but because it was the front side of the fence, I didn't have anywhere to put my feet, and I wasn't tall enough to get over the fence otherwise. By the time I figured out that I couldn't get over the fence the same way, Maggie was right behind me.

I knew what was going on in the house at that moment. One or more of the girls had heard Maggie barking and were on the way out. I had maybe 30 seconds before someone came outside and retaliated. It wasn't enough time to execute the plan, especially with Maggie on my tail.

I knew that right next to the house was a little side gate led directly into my yard. I knew I could get to that side gate with the time I had left and get back to my house before anyone saw me, so I bolted!

I side-stepped Maggie and headed straight for the house. The whole length of the yard, I could feel her breath on my leg. As I got closer to the house, I saw August running into the sunroom. We locked eyes for just a second, and I started to panic because nothing was going according to plan. In the heat of the moment, I opened the gate and ran out of their yard. I didn't realize until it was too late that Maggie had gotten out also.

"Oh no!" I mumbled to myself when I realized what had happened. I watched in horror as Maggie started to run. I dove to try to catch her, but she wriggled free from my grasp.

"Mitchell!" August screamed, "Why did you let her out?!"

"I didn't mean to!" I replied.

"Yeah right," she said, rolling her eyes.

Her annoyance did tempt me to start a fight, but I did feel guilty about Maggie getting out. "Look," I said seriously, "I get that we're not friends anymore, but Maggie is gonna get hit by a car if we don't do something right now. What do you want me to do to help?"

"Go inside the house," August said after thinking about it for a second, "tell the girls what's going on and grab dog treats."

I ran to the back door and entered the sunroom. Aspen saw me from the living room.

"Mitchell what are you doing in here!" she yelled as she ran towards me.

"Maggie got out and August told me to come in and get help and grab dog treats!"

Aspen stopped in her tracks. "How did she get out?"

"It was my fault, but I'm trying to help now. Please tell me where the dog treats are!"

"I'll grab them," she said, reluctantly accepting my help. "You get the other girls!"

I gathered Arden and Lo-lo, and the four of us ran into the front yard to meet up with August. "Where is she?" Arden asked.

"She was right here when I left her!" I replied.

"Look," Lo-lo said, "she's running up the street."

"Let's go!" Aspen exclaimed, running after August.

Now at the top of the street, there was a Methodist Church and an adjoining funeral home. Directly behind the church was a little park. In the middle of the park was a giant white gazebo, and next to that was a fenced-in children's playground. About 3/4 of the way up the street, an alley leads directly to the children's playground.

Maggie was about to run off of Meadow Park Drive and right into the middle of traffic. The last chance we had to catch her would be if we could divert Maggie to the playground.

"Aspen," Arden exclaimed, "you and Lo-lo catch up to August and get her into the church parking lot! Mitchell, grab the treats and come with me!"

Everyone agreed, and Arden and I ran down the alley. Arden was a lot faster than me, so she got to the playground first. By the time I caught up, I saw the other three girls chasing Maggie around the parking lot. "Mitchell, give me the treats and hold this gate open!" Arden told me, "Once Maggie is inside, close it!"

"Yes ma'am!" I said enthusiastically, handing over the treats.

"Maggie! Maggie!" Arden called, ignoring me.

Maggie heard Arden, looked over, and recognized the treats. Arden lured her towards me and walked inside the playground. As instructed, when Maggie walked in, I closed the gate behind her!

CHAPTER 30: THE FAIRYTALE DREAMER
03/14/2011-03/15/2011

"**Y**ES!" August, Aspen, and Lo-lo exclaimed in unison. They hugged each other, and I went to join.

"Ummm, what are you doing?" Aspen asked.

"Oh… sorry I thought--"

"Mitchell," August interjected, "Thank you for helping us get Maggie back, but you're the reason that she got out in the first place, and you still hurt us by lying."

"But, I'm sorry!" I screamed, "I just helped you, why is it not--"

"Because sometimes Mitchell, sorry just isn't good enough!" August yelled back.

I turned around and looked at Arden, who was petting Maggie. We made eye contact, and immediately she looked at the ground. "Fine!" I said, walking away, "Be that way!"

I stalked back home, trying not to cry. When I got back, I saw Greg standing in my front yard. When he saw me, he stretched his arms out dramatically and said, "What the heck happened?"

"Oh my gosh, I am so sorry man! Maggie got out and we had to chase her!"

I knew Greg was mad, but when he realized I was upset, he asked me what was wrong. I told him what had happened, and we went to his house where we talked things out and planned our next move.

***

"... And then he went in for a hug!" Aspen exclaimed at dinner that night, "Can you believe that?"

"What's so unbelievable about that?" Rich asked.

"What do you mean 'what's so unbelievable about that'?!" August countered, stunned.

"I mean, why is that surprising? You guys were friends a week ago. He spent more time with you guys then I ever did with any of my friends, when I was his age. Do you really want to throw that away?"

"Dad," Arden argued, "we put all the effort we had into that relationship, but he still lied to us! We're not throwing this relationship away, he did that. All we are doing is defending ourselves, so we don't get hurt again."

Rich looked at his other three daughters, who were all nodding in agreement. That night Rich couldn't get to sleep because he was worried about my relationship with the girls. He got out of bed, walked downstairs and got on the computer. He said a quick prayer asking God to help him find something to explain this to the girls, and God answered.

Rich found a blog post about children with Asperger's called, "Lying or Wishful Thinking: Which one is your youngster doing?" The author states, "For these special needs kids, it may be helpful to think less in terms of 'lying' and more in terms of 'wishful thinking' (i.e., they often say what they would like to be true, rather than what is clearly and objectively true)."

After reading the blog, Rich realized what was going on. I wasn't lying out of malice; I was lying because I wished that the girls were my friends. The next day as the girls were getting ready for school, Rich told them about his findings. By doing this, Rich started an argument with the girls, that would go on for about a month. While she tried to ignore his points, eventually, Rich began to get to Arden.

The reason for this was that Arden has a heart of gold and I had a special place in that heart. Because we grew up in such an intimate friendship, even though everything inevitably fell apart, Arden looked back on our fairytale childhood with incredible fondness. So, despite how betrayed she felt because I lied, she wanted things to be the way they were during the fairytale, or at least the way things were while we were recording *Miracle Child.*

CHAPTER 31: THE GINKGO TREE

03/18/2011

A spring/summertime hangout for the girls was a ginkgo tree located in "The Circle." Every year at the beginning of spring, the Anderson girls would tie a circular green swing up on the ginkgo tree as well as long ropes to help them climb. The following Friday, after Maggie got out, they did just that.

Mom drove me home from school, and as we pulled around "The Circle", I saw August, Arden, Aspen, Lo-lo, Shelby, and Melody in the act of setting up the swing. I got a massive grin on my face, and I started to flap my hands.

"What's up?" Mom asked.

"It's nothing." I said, pulling out my phone.

I went inside, ran to my room, and called Greg. I told him that it was happening and that it was time to execute our next plan. We met in my front yard and waited for Lo-lo to get off the swing and give it to one of the other girls. As soon as she got off, I grabbed the swing and jumped on.

"Get off!" August yelled from the tree.

"Why?" I replied with a sly smile.

"Because it's our swing!" The Anderson girls replied.

"Well technically," Greg pointed out, "'The Circle' is city property and by extension so is the ginkgo tree.

You might own the swing, but because the city owns the tree, anyone can use the swing."

"'Well technically'," Melody mocked her brother, "they don't have to keep that swing out here, they can always bring it to their property!"

"Yeah!" The Anderson girls cheered.

"Okay, if that's what you want." I said, hopping off the swing.

"And just so you guys can't climb the tree," August said after she untied the swing, "we're going to take our ropes too!"

So, Greg and I watched as they took everything off the tree and dragged them to the Andersons' house. "Have a nice day!" Greg called as they walked away. The girls looked back and glared at us, and we just smiled back.

We stood in the circle for a while, waiting for one of the girls to look out the window. Eventually, as expected, Lo-lo and Shelby did. When we noticed that they were watching us, I clasped my hands together and hoisted Greg to reach the first branch. I couldn't hold him long enough, though, and he fell.

Greg then attempted to climb the tree on his own. After three or four attempts, he managed to hang upside down under the first branch, put his legs on top of the branch, and flip himself so that he was on top. I tried to copy him next, but I was not coordinated enough to pull it off. "Maybe instead of hanging under and then flipping yourself," Greg suggested, "Grab the first branch, pull yourself up and put your arm over the top, and then reach for the second branch and get on top."

I did as he instructed, and after about 15 minutes, I succeeded. When I was finally in the tree, Greg and I looked at the Andersons' house. Staring out the window in shock were all of the girls. We smiled victoriously, knowing that we had just taken away their haven.

CHAPTER 32: THE SCATTERBALL GAME
03/21/2011-04/15/2011

While in Derek's class the following Monday, Derek handed out blue invitations to everybody.

"What are these?" I asked.

"They're invitations to a prom for kids on the spectrum that will be held next month at Longmoore High School!"

The dance became the talk of the school that day. At lunchtime, I sat alone because I was avoiding people since I still felt terrible about the whole Caroline thing.

"Hey Mitch!" Zach said, sitting across the table from me.

"Hey man. How are you?"

"I'm doing well. So Caroline, Jake, myself, and a few others and I are going to this prom, and I was wondering if you wanted to come with us."

"Thanks dude!" I said, trying to avoid eye contact, "But I don't think it's a good idea… still kinda awkward, you know?"

"Yeah, but it's a month away. By that time, I'm sure it will all be smoothed over, and if not, maybe you going is what fixes it."

I wanted to start an argument with Zach because I knew he didn't understand how much Jake hated me for what had happened, and why he was right to do so. But I knew he was trying to help, and he was trying to include me, and I did want to go, so I agreed.

***

The next month went by with nothing major to note. I would go to school, feel guilty about the Caroline situation, and then go home and torment the girls with Greg. I think it started to take a toll on Greg, though, because the more we fought with the girls, the more the girls disliked him, and the farther away his chances with August got. Everything came to a head the day before the prom.

Once dinner had ended on that fateful Friday night, I checked my phone and saw that I had a text from Greg. He asked if my brothers and I would like to play Scatterball.

The best way to describe the game Scatterball is every man for himself dodgeball. It was a game that Greg would play with his church group. The rules are simple:

1. At the beginning of the game, someone throws one ball up, yells, "scatter," and a ball has to hit the ground three times before anyone can grab it

2. When you have the ball, you can only take three steps before you have to throw it.

3. Once you get hit, you are out, and you have to sit down where you were hit.

4. If you throw the ball and somebody catches it, you are out.

5. After you get out and you're sitting down, if the ball comes to you, you can pick it up, stand up, throw the ball, and if you hit someone, they are out, and you are back in.

6. The last person standing wins.

7. Scatterball Revenge: Scatterball Revenge is the same game with all the previous rules, except if the

person who got you out gets out by anyone, then you are back in. Scatterball Revenge is the version that we usually played because it's more interesting.

I asked the boys if they wanted to play Scatterball with Greg, and they agreed.

We walked out to Greg's yard and started to play. We played three games in 30 minutes, and Greg came out on top every time. Because he wanted a little more of a challenge and presumably because he wanted to mend the bridge between himself and August, he made a suggestion.

"I think we should invite the girls to play!"

"NO!" I exclaimed, without a second of hesitation, "We're not friends, they don't get to play with us!"

"Mitchell," Greg said calmly, "It's more fun with more people anyway, it's just a game, it doesn't mean everything is okay!"

"But, it's just--"

"No Mitchell!" he continued firmly, "they're playing with us! Ryan, go get them."

Ryan left and returned with the Anderson girls and Shelby while Greg went inside and got Melody. Greg explained the rules, while the girls and I glared at each other.

"Scatter," Greg yelled. The ball bounced once, twice, and on the third time, I ran for it. Aspen was the closest person to me, so I launched it at her and got her out. To get Aspen back in the game, the remaining five girls tried to get me out.

Every time I would get out, Ryan or Greg would get the girl who got me out to get me back in. However, as soon as I would get back in, another girl would get me out. It got to the point where they would break the rules (take more than three steps or move from where they got out) to get me out. Eventually, August hit me in the face with the ball, and I lost it.

I charged and tackled her, and she hit the ground hard. "Mitchell, stop!" Greg yelled, pulling me up by my arm.
I suddenly became very angry with Greg. He was supposed to be my friend; he was supposed to be loyal to me! He wasn't supposed to be taking her side!

"Why?" I growled at him, "Because you *love* her?"

CHAPTER 33: THE BRICK
04/15/2011-04/16/2011

Greg immediately blushed. August stood up and looked at him. Everyone just stood there for what felt like an eternity, not sure what to do next. Eventually, Greg walked back into his house, and everyone else slowly left until it was just me.

The next day I stayed inside until about 4:30 p.m. because I felt awkward about the events of the night before. Around that time, I looked out the window and saw Greg climbing the ginkgo tree.

"Hey man," I said awkwardly as I walked up to the tree.

"Hey." he replied dryly.

"Dude, I'm really sorry about last night."

"Why did you do that? I told you about that in confidence!"

"I know. I just got really angry and I felt like you were choosing their side, and I made a mistake."

"Mitchell I really don't know what to tell you. Yes, of course I forgive you and I know you're going through a lot right now with the girls, but it's just too much drama man. I can't do it anymore."

"What do you mean?" I asked.

"Do whatever you want to get back at the girls but count me out of it."

Of course, I understood why he wanted out, but I was furious about it, specifically with the girls. If they hadn't been singling me out the whole game, I would not have attacked August, Greg wouldn't have pulled me off her, and I wouldn't have spilled his secret out of rage. This situation was their fault!

At that moment, I decided that before I went to the prom, I would annoy the girls. I ran into my backyard and saw Dad and Pop-pop sitting on the back porch. I made sure they didn't see me, and then I hopped the Andersons' fence. Coincidentally, I landed right next to a brick with a rope tied around it. The rope was short, but it had enough length to swing the brick around. I decided that I could claim that the girls were planning to use the brick as a weapon.

"Hey!" Arden called from the back porch, "What are you doing here?!" I grabbed the brick and ran, as Arden and Aspen chased after me.

"Dad, Dad!" I called as I ran towards my backyard, "Look what I found!"

"What's going on?" he asked.

"The girls made a weapon and they were going to use it on us!"

"What?" he continued as he hopped down the stairs on his crutches. I explained the situation, and when I had finished, Dad called Arden and Aspen over.

"What happened?"

"Well," Arden explained, "we were sitting on our deck, and we looked over and we saw Mitchell in our yard. The only thing we did was chase him out of our yard!"

"Okay!" I retorted. "Yeah, you didn't do anything right now, but how do you explain the brick?! Why would you have a brick with a rope around it if you weren't going to use it as a weapon?!"

"Oh, come on Mitchell!" Aspen exclaimed, "That is crap, and you know it!"

At this, I started yelling at the girls. "SURE OKAY! WHO IS HE GOING TO BELIEVE, HIS SON OR THE GOOD FOR NOTHING GIRLS WHO SPEND ALL THEIR TIME--"

"MITCHELL!" Dad yelled, "STOP!" He took a breath and continued, "Go inside, I will handle this."

"But Dad--"

"GO!"

I dropped the brick and turned around to go inside. I saw Pop-pop standing on the deck, watching everything unfold. I avoided eye contact with him as I went inside and ran to my room. About 5 minutes later, my door opened, and Dad walked through.

"What was that about?"

"What do you mean? I told you what happened!" I said between tears.

"No, I mean why did you yell at them like that?"

"Cuz they are mean people!"

"Mitchell, whose side do you think I'm on, theirs or yours?"

"Mine."

"Then let me handle it, okay? That wasn't your place to yell at them."

I wanted to tell him it was my place because they had hurt me, but Mom walked in before I got the chance.

"Hey, guys sorry to interrupt." She said.

"No, you're fine." Dad replied, "What's up?"

"Well, it's 5:00, Mitchell, and I have to drop you off at 6:00 at Zach's house."

"Okay," Dad said, "we'll talk about this later, get dressed."

CHAPTER 34: THE PROM
04/16/2011

Mom drove me to Zach's house after I put on a nice suit and a bow tie, and she got a few pictures. Mom dropped me off at his house, I knocked on the door, and Zach opened it. We walked into the kitchen where Jake, Caroline, a few other people from Haugland that I didn't personally know, and Zach's mom were waiting. Zach's mom and I caught up as I hadn't seen her in almost a year. I glanced at Caroline and noticed that there was something wrong, but I could not figure out what it was.

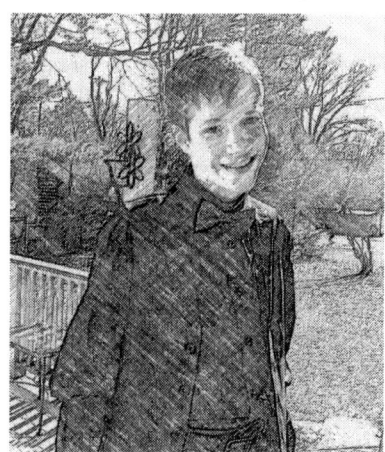

When we got to Longmoore High School, a student took us to the gym. The gym had maybe 200 to 300 people dancing around. We walked up to the sign-in table and were given name tags. The students in charge of planning this prom had set up a sign-up sheet online. One of the questions was along the lines of, "Is the student attending in a relationship?" The reason for this was so one of the teens, who helped set up the prom, could be paired with a single autistic student so that they wouldn't feel left out. The girl I got paired with was approximately 16 or 17 years old.

You have to understand, at this point, I was 13 years old. I had just recently hit puberty, and I was currently suffering from major acne. On the other hand, this girl was on the cusp of adulthood. She didn't have any acne, and even if she had, it wouldn't have mattered because she was ridiculously attractive. I think it's safe to say that I felt a little underprepared.

"Hi!" she said, smiling and extending her hand, "My name is Natalie!"

"Umm, hello," I replied, shaking her hand. "My name is Mitch."

"Nice to meet you Mitch," Natalie said. "Do you want to dance?"

"Sure." I said hesitantly. She took my hand in hers as we walked into the crowd of people. The song was a high-energy song, so everyone was jumping around. Natalie was dancing and trying to hype me up, but I was just a little too confused to get into it, and she noticed.

"Are you okay?" She asked.

"Yeah, I'm fine," I said. "I've just never been in this situation before."

"What do you mean?"

"Danced with a girl that is as pretty as you… Well, I've never danced with any girl really!"

She let out a chuckle, "Well, that's okay! I can help you get comfortable with it."

"Really?"

"Yeah sure, I mean you're going to do it eventually; you may as well get practice."

"That's true--"

"So, here's the deal," she explained, "they play a fast-paced song, and then play a slow dance song, so the next song is slow."

"Okay, what do I do?"

"You're going to put your hands here," She said, placing them on her waist, "and I'll place mine here," and she put her hands on my shoulders.

We danced for about an hour, going back and forth between fast and slow songs. Eventually, while we were dancing to a slow song, Natalie whispered in my ear, "Who is that girl that's watching us?"

I turned around and saw Caroline looking at us. When we made eye contact, she turned away and walked out of the gym.

"No one… just a girl from school."

Natalie raised her eyebrow just as the slow song ended, and a fast one began. She was curious, but she decided not to dig too deeply into the issue. "I don't know about you," Natalie said, "but I'm thirsty. Do you want to get some punch?"

We walked up to the punch table and got our drinks. We went off to the side to drink, and Jake walked up to us. "Hey Mitch, can we talk?"

"You've made it pretty clear you don't want to talk to me."

"Yeah, cuz you kissed my girlfriend!"

Natalie looked at me, confused. "I didn't say it wasn't justified," I said.

"Look," he said, "Caroline and I broke up the other day. We got in a fight and I think she likes you. I still want to be friends with you, I was just kind of mad about everything that happened. Would you be okay if we went back to the way things were?"

"Yeah, of course!" I said.

"Thank you!" he said as he walked away.

"So, that girl," Natalie asked, "The one that was watching us, was that Caroline?"

"Maybe."

"Well, are you going to go talk to her?"

"It's complicated."

"Why?"

I decided I needed to explain everything to Natalie.

"Oh my gosh!" Natalie exclaimed when I had finished. "Mitch, you have to tell her!"

"You think she would be okay with that?"

"If she likes you as much as it looks like she does, that will not be a problem and maybe she can help you move on!"

I smiled and walked out the same door that Caroline had. I found myself in the school hallway, and I saw Caroline leaning up against the wall. I sat down next to her. "Hi," I said.

"What do you want?"

"That girl I told you about wasn't my girlfriend. I wanted her to be, but she wasn't."

"Then, why did you say she was?"

"I thought it would make things easier to cope with if I pretended, she was, because then she would have known how I felt."

"Well, it doesn't matter if she knew before she moved, you'll see her again and you can tell her then."

"No, I can't. She didn't just move, she passed away almost two years ago."

"What!"

"Yeah. It was the hardest thing I've ever had to go through."

"Why are you telling me this?"

"Because I don't want to make the same mistake with you."

"Mitch, I'm not dying."

"No!" I exclaimed, realizing my mistake. "I mean, I don't want you to not know how I feel about you. Last summer right after everything happened, I told my friend Elizabeth everything. It's kind of a long story, but basically, she told me that my life was going to get better. I didn't really believe her at first, but then I met you. You make me feel so happy. I think Elizabeth was right, my life is going to get better because of you."

"Oh, Jake talked to you, didn't he?"

"He might have said a few things. Do you want to dance?"

"Sure." She giggled.

I took her hand in mine, and we walked back into the gym. Natalie saw us walking together, and she smiled and gave me a thumbs up. A slow song was playing, so I showed her how to dance to it, and we swayed to the music. When the song ended, I leaned in and kissed her!

CHAPTER 35: THE BROKEN DISK

04/16/2011-04/18/2011

"**S**URE OKAY! WHO IS HE GOING TO BELIEVE, HIS SON OR THE GOOD FOR NOTHING GIRLS WHO SPEND ALL THEIR TIME--"

"MITCHELL!" Dad yelled, "STOP!" He took a breath and continued, "Go inside, I will handle this."

"But Dad--"

"GO!"

I dropped the brick and turned around to go inside. After I left, Dad gave the girls a minor scolding. It wasn't too big of a deal because the whole brick incident was stupid, but the girls were still mad because I got them in trouble.

"He's a jerk!" August said about me when Arden and Aspen told her and Lo-lo what had happened.

"What do you think we should do?" Aspen asked.

August thought about it for a second, then smiled and said, "I know exactly what we'll do!"

***

I woke up the next morning on a high! I couldn't believe what had happened the night before. Even though I wasn't sure what our relationship status was, I had a pretty good guess. I decided to talk to Caroline about it the next day at school.

When we got home from church, I walked upstairs and took off my "Sunday best" in favor of something more comfortable. While I was still changing, I heard a knock at the door.

"Mitchell," Luke said, running up the stairs, "the girls are outside, they want to see you!"

Confused, I went outside. All four of the Anderson girls stood in my front yard. When she saw me, August stepped forward and handed me the disc. "Here you go!" She said with a smile that, in retrospect, was fake. But I didn't realize it at the time. I was too excited!

I ran back inside, turned on the TV, popped the movie in the DVD player, and hit play. After about 30 seconds, I realized that this wasn't the same disc that we originally made. The girls had blurred out every scene in which any of them appeared!

I stormed outside, furious, and I started yelling at the girls. I don't remember what I said exactly; I only remember screaming so loud that my throat hurt. Pop-pop heard me screaming from inside, came outside, picked me up, and brought me back into the house. When I got inside, I ran to my room and stayed there for the rest of the day.

Around 8:00 or 9:00 that night, I came back downstairs because I was starving. Pop-pop and Dad were sitting in the living room and saw me come downstairs. They asked me to sit down so we could talk. When I did, Dad asked me what had happened, and I explained the situation.

"Mitchell," Pop-pop said, "you can't react like that."

"Why?"

"It would be like giving someone who doesn't like you, more ammunition for the guns they already possess."

"So, what should I do?"

"You should ignore them. Then they won't have any ammo," Dad said.

After this, the conversation repeated itself for roughly 15 minutes. As the discussion wore on, Pop-pop started to think something along the lines of *Mitchell definitely understands why he shouldn't react that way. It's completely logical, and he has virtually admitted that he understands. So why is he still fighting us on this?*

He followed this train of thought, and it led him to the only logical explanation, "Do you still want to be friends with the girls?" Pop-pop asked

"No!" I lied, not very convincingly.

"Mitchell--" Dad said, catching my lie.

"Okay fine! Maybe I do, but it doesn't matter. Not like they actually want to be my friend anymore."

"You guys have grown up together," Dad said, "and you just recently spent a ton of time together. I'm sure they still would like to be friends. You just have to make an effort!"

I went to bed that night with a new goal in mind: Become friends with the girls and fix our problems. The next day after school, I waited in the circle for someone to come outside. At one point, I saw Barbara drive "Old Betsy" up the street with August and Aspen in the car. Three minutes later, Arden came outside, walking Maggie.

CHAPTER 36: THE GREATTASTIC ADVENTURERS

04/18/2011

Arden saw me and avoided eye contact. She started to walk up the street, and I followed her. "Hey," I said, "can we talk?" She ignored me. "I know you're mad at me, but I really want to be friends with you guys again."

"Ha!" she said sarcastically, "Okay!"

"I'm serious!"

"Sure! Can you leave me alone please?"

"No! Arden, can you at least hear me out?"

"After what you did, what could you possibly say, that could ever lead me, lead us to ever trust you again?"

"First of all, I'm sorry I lied to you, but I only did it because I didn't know how to ask you guys to be my friends. You guys hated me for so long before Miracle Child, what was I supposed to do, tell you the truth and risk you guys saying no?"

"We 'hated you' because you bullied us!"

"I did not! You guys bullied me!"

"Mitchell, you called us names, hit us, and lied about things that we never did, just to get us in trouble! How are we supposed to react?"

As soon as she said that, my entire perspective on the situation shifted. I thought I was the victim. I had thought that they were ignoring me because they didn't understand autism and thought I was weird. While not understanding autism did add to the problem, my actions caused the girls to dislike me.

"Oh my gosh--" I said, taking a pause, "I'm so sorry, I never saw it like that. I promise I'll make it better, just please give me another chance."

Arden thought about it for a second. Her father's words echoed in her head: *You guys were friends a week ago. He spent more time with you guys than I ever did with any of my friends when I was his age. Do you want to throw that away?*

No, she didn't want to throw it away. As I stated before, she wanted the group to go back to how it was while we were recording Miracle Child. This moment was her chance to make that happen. "Okay," she said, smiling, "I forgive you, and I'm sorry for making you feel like you had to lie to become our friend."

I smiled back at her excitedly that things were about to go back to normal. We didn't know it at the time, but this decision would eventually transform the sisterhood into something completely new. So new, in fact, that we would give it a new name: The Greattastic Adventurers!

CHAPTER 37: THE BEGINNING
04/18/2011-04/19/2011

"**W**hat do we do now?" I asked Arden as we were heading home from the walk.

"Well, you made up with me, but you still need to apologize to the others. That's going to be a little harder."

"Yeah, I can imagine."

"Well, you're in luck," Arden said. "My mom took August and Aspen to the store and they should be gone for about 20 more minutes. But Lo-lo and Shelby are home. If you apologize to them, when you apologize to the other two, we can all back you up."

When we got to the house, we walked into the TV room and found Lo-lo and Shelby sitting on the couch. "What are you doing here?" Shelby asked incredulously.

"Guys," Arden said, "Mitchie has something to tell you."

"Arlo," I said, "I'm really sorry that I hurt you and your sisters. I was struggling to understand a lot of things that were happening with you guys, and, umm I really hope that we can be friends again. And Shelby, I'm really sorry that I told you about Lo-lo avoiding you. I shouldn't have done that, that was mean-spirited and unnecessary. Can you guys forgive me?"

"Mitchell, how can I trust you," Lo-lo asked, "after you lied to us?"

"Lo-lo," Arden said, "August lied to you. You don't have a sister named Susie. But you still trust August, right?"

After she recuperated from the shock of learning that Susie wasn't real, Lo-lo said, "Yes, but that's different!"

"No, it's not I mean, one was more of a joke, but a lie is a lie. I think he deserves a second chance!" Lo-lo agreed, just as Rich came downstairs. We all talked until Barbara, August and Aspen returned.

"What's going on?" August yelled.

"Mitchell is going to stay for dinner," Rich said. "He needs to talk to you guys."

At dinner, we sat down, and I apologized to August and Aspen. As expected, they weren't very receptive to it. "We are not going to forgive you!" August said. "You've hurt us too much!"

"Yeah!" Aspen echoed.

These comments led to an argument that lasted the entire dinner, which ended in me getting discouraged. In a huff, I left the house and started to walk home. Before I got to the end of the driveway, Rich caught up to me.

"Mitchell," he said, "just hang on. I know it looks like things aren't going to work out right now, but just give them a little time. I promise they will come around!"

I thanked him for his kind words, even though I didn't believe him, and I went home. I walked inside, went upstairs, brushed my teeth, and crawled into my bed, defeated.

***

The next day after school, I grabbed an after-school snack and started walking around the house. As I was walking around, I looked out the window, and I froze. August was walking towards my house. When she saw me standing in the window, she smiled and motioned for me to come outside. And that was just the beginning...

EPILOGUE: RULES FOR A GREATTASTIC LIFE

The first draft of this book started with me getting ready to go to college. I planned to tell the "Miracle Child" story, along with some things that happened after, through flashbacks. There was a problem with writing a book this way, however. I couldn't create a present-day timeline because I didn't know how that story would end. After a year of writing the book that way and running into a ton of story-related complications, I decided to delete the whole thing and write a story about my childhood.

I still thought the college/adult stuff was interesting, so I decided to start a blog called "Rules for a Greattastic Life" as a supplement. I immediately became an Autism advocate and decided to use the blog to talk about autistic adulthood struggles.

A year after I started the blog, Mom shared one of my posts, and a family friend commented, "So when can we hear Mitchell read his blogs? I hear his voice (when I read it), but I would love to hear his voice reading his own blogs on my way to work." That comment led me to start a podcast as an extension to the blog.

If you would like to follow my story and stay up to date on my future projects, you can find me on Instagram @rulesforagreattastic and other social media as Rules for a Greattastic Life.

Have a Greattastic Day and Be Safe!

J. Mitchell Ulibarri

ABOUT THE AUTHOR

John "Mitchell" Ulibarri is both the author and host of a blog and podcast called "Rules for a Greattastic Life" about his life on the autism spectrum. He is a native to Columbus, Ohio and enjoys going on adventures with his friends and family.

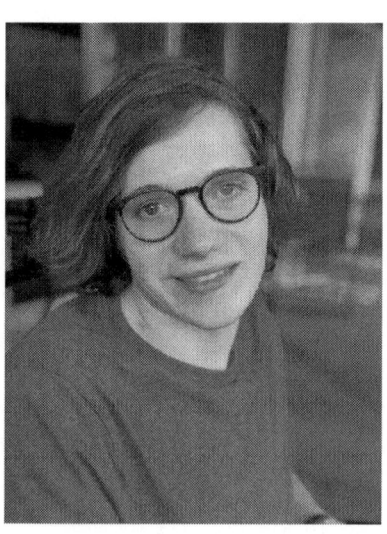

Made in the USA
Middletown, DE
28 May 2023

30906014R00099